FIREBREATHER
FITNESS

T0244015

FIREBREATHER FITNESS

Work Your Body, Mind, and Spirit into the Best Shape of Your Life

GREG AMUNDSON

WITH T. J. MURPHY

VELO.
press.

an imprint of Ulysses Press
PO Box 3440
Berkeley, CA 93703
www.velopress.com

VeloPress is the leading publisher of books on sports for passionate and dedicated athletes
around the world. Focused on cycling, triathlon, running, swimming, nutrition/diet, and
more, VeloPress books help you achieve your goals and reach the top of your game.

ISBN: 978-1-64604-797-0

Cover design: Peter Garceau
Photos: Jeff Clark, pp. 24–77, 194–202, 205, 258; courtesy of Greg Amundson, front cover,
   pp. 5, 88, 99, 129, 151, 156, 168, 184; Jason Innes, p. 85 (top); Grasseto/Thinkstock, p. 85
   (bottom); Scott Draper, p. 259; David Leys, back cover
Art direction: Vicki Hopewell

Printed in the United States of America
10 9 8 7 6 5 4 3 2 1

This book is dedicated in loving memory to my mom and dad, who inspired me from a young age to pursue a "heart like Christ" and to develop my mind, body, and spirit in such a way that I could better serve others.

CONTENTS

SPIRIT

PLANS

STANDARDS

Foreword

I first met Greg Amundson in 2007, at a CrossFit Level 1 certification with founder Greg Glassman. He was an impressive individual, to say the least. Greg's Firebreather performance, his example, and his commitment to teaching helped to inspire the first generations of CrossFitters (including myself) who were opening the first wave of CrossFit affiliates around the world.

What many don't know about Greg is what drives him to train and teach with such mad-dog intensity: a commitment to serve others. During his years with Coach Glassman in Santa Cruz, California, and at his own gym, CrossFit Amundson, Greg was also a full-time law-enforcement officer on a journey that led to him becoming a SWAT officer and later a DEA special agent and Army captain.

Greg was—and is—both an athlete and a warrior. He doesn't train to look better in a pair of jeans, but rather to be better prepared for his job and to put his life on the line to protect others. So it did not surprise me to find out that Greg was intrigued with my SEALFIT warrior development training. I have long believed that to reach your true potential, you must embark upon integrated training of the body, mind, emotions, intuition, and spirit. This process, which is delivered in our SEALFIT Kokoro and Unbeatable Mind trainings, helps to develop a serious passion for life. It also simplifies things, helping you to focus with a laser-like intensity on your main purpose and mission in life. When you tap into this potential, you access individual capacities of self-discipline, mental toughness, stamina, and endurance that otherwise remain untapped.

I enjoyed watching Greg lead his class through the 53-hour Kokoro Camp number 12 at SEALFIT. While Kokoro is certainly an incredible physical struggle, the challenge goes way beyond the physical, testing character and spirit. One of the ultimate lessons you learn there is that resiliency and leadership are not about you, but the team. You have your breakthrough moment at Kokoro when you stop thinking about your own pity party and start focusing on serving your teammates.

As I watched Greg lead, I saw immediately that he already embodied this truth. His attitude of service and humility never let up as he navigated the event and gave his all to help those who were struggling. As a former SEAL commander who has deployed to combat and led the nation's most elite warriors, I knew then that Greg Amundson was someone who had my back, and that of anyone else he was in service to.

I am excited to see Greg revealing his servant philosophy and full-dimension training ideas to the world. The book you hold in your hands reveals powerful truths about achieving optimal performance. While getting in a hard workout will help you burn body fat and build muscle, there's simply no realizing the complete set of gifts and capacities you were born with unless you give similar attention to your mental and spiritual depths.

There's a reason why Greg has had the tenacity to train as hard as he does, year in, year out. It is grounded in his commitment to serve others, which he has built into a set of rituals and exercises that feeds his soul and allows him to wake up every day excited to give everything he has. Greg's passion for integrating mind, body, and spirit through his holistic training program is inspiring, and can be a catalyst for you to do the same.

I encourage you to read Greg's book carefully and implement his strategies. The world needs you to be your best self, and Greg is ready to help you. The time to start is now!

MARK DIVINE
US Navy SEALs Commander (Ret.),
SEALFIT founder, and New York Times best-selling author of
The Way of the SEAL and Unbeatable Mind

Introduction

Seventeen years ago, I launched myself into a career of protection and service in the law-enforcement profession. It would prove to be a journey of great discovery that would diverge into different challenges. I would ultimately serve as each of the following during different stages of my life: deputy sheriff, SWAT operator, sniper, US Army captain, DEA special agent, and DEA liaison to the Border Enforcement Security Task Force (BEST) team.

Throughout this period, I was relentlessly developing, experimenting with, and sharpening my training. My work as a first responder and military leader became my live-action testing grounds. Each day that I put on a uniform and prepared for a duty shift, my day was like a blank piece of paper. I had no clue of when, where, and what situations and problems I might be called to. However, I did expect to face situations that tested my capacity to make sound decisions in a split second. To cope with that stress and meet those challenges effectively, I needed to be able to draw on my most important assets: my mind, my body, and my spirit.

My body was primed. As an early participant in CrossFit, today a global movement in physical conditioning, I had seen remarkable physical gains, using old-school movements such as push-ups, pull-ups, squats, and kettlebell swings, mixing them up constantly into circuit workouts that encouraged high-intensity efforts. I felt on top of my physical game.

But it wasn't enough. I knew that I needed to do more than just develop my physical body if I wanted to thrive in a warrior profession and continue improving. I felt strongly that in order to achieve my full potential, I needed to integrate my training, developing not only my body but also my mind and spirit. Over the next several years, exploring various techniques and disciplines, working with world-class coaches and mentors, and experimenting on my own, I honed a set of mental, physical, and spiritual tools, which I infused into a fully integrated training program.

Firebreather Fitness was born.

This holistic, integrated approach has enabled my continued performance improvements for 16 years and counting. In fact, today I'm training harder than I ever have in my life. I continue to accrue gains in my physical, mental, and spiritual capacities. And rather than burning out or getting stale, I am as fired up about it as I have ever been! My enthusiasm to train hard is greater than ever, and I can't wait to wake up tomorrow and do it all again. This is the reason for this book. I want to share that zeal with others who are interested in giving everything they've got to achieve everything they can.

As this book unfolds, I will dig deeply into the physical, mental, and spiritual components of the program. But I think a great place to begin is by sharing with you my initial steps into a Firebreather Fitness approach.

MY FIRST EXPERIENCE in law enforcement began in the summer of 1999 at the Ray Simon Criminal Justice Training Center in Modesto, California, as a reserve police officer recruit for Scotts Valley Police Department. Two years later, I was hired as a deputy sheriff with the Santa Cruz County Sheriff's Office, and started another police academy, this time at the South Bay Regional Law Enforcement Training Academy, in San Jose, California. The physical training at both academies was conventional at the time, consisting of long-distance formation runs and bodybuilding workouts three times per week.

Runs were aerobic—no sprinting—and because we ran in platoon formation, the runs were at the pace of the slowest member of the group, not the fastest. The bodybuilding training was the kind of thing you might see promoted on the cover of a newsstand magazine, selling readers on bigger biceps and rock-hard abs. A workout might be three sets of eight exercises using weight machines, like lat pull-downs and leg extensions. We did eight to twelve repetitions per set, with ample rest between sets. Bodybuilding sessions took place on days we were not running. We never lifted to the point of exhaustion. These were routines designed to maximize muscle size, not develop power or stamina.

We also practiced defensive tactics and firearms, although never on days that we exercised. I wonder now, why wouldn't you practice these kinds of skills on a day when you are tired from conditioning? Wouldn't that be more like the real thing? Shouldn't you simulate firearm accuracy and defensive tactics when your heart rate is over 200 beats per minute because of a fight or foot chase? Or both?

I never considered this gaping fault in the academy program. I bought into what the police academy trainers were telling me and assumed cable-crossovers and biceps curls would prepare me for the demands of the job.

After graduating from the academy, I was partnered with a field-training officer (FTO). The FTO's job is to help you transition your new police skills from the controlled confines of the academy to the less predictable nature of the real world.

I was in the first week of my field training when my training was put to the test. I was apprehending a parolee who decided he was up for a battle. The fight started and we quickly went down to the ground—it was both a wrestling match and a battle of wills.

It quickly became apparent that I wasn't physically prepared for an all-out street fight. I felt like I was breathing through a straw. My heart pounded wildly and I was gasping for air. I tried to produce a forceful punch or throw, but the muscles I'd supposedly been training felt lifeless.

The truth hit: I wasn't ready for the harsh reality of the job. The training had failed me. In an impromptu fight with a random parolee, I could barely hang on.

If all I could do was hang on in the first confrontation that I experienced as a young deputy sheriff, just out of the academy at a time when I was in peak shape, how was I going to be able to do my job well as I grew older? How was I going to be able to serve and protect the public, as well as my comrades in the law-enforcement profession? At what risk was this lack of preparation putting both myself and others? The line of work that I was choosing was literally putting my life on the line. I knew that I had to match the critical nature of my job with an equally critical form of training.

I went seeking advice and got some from local martial artist and long-time friend Sam Radetsky of Santa Cruz, California. He told me about a "crazy coach, doing crazy workouts, inside a crazy little gym in the corner of a Brazilian jiu-jitsu place." His description alone piqued my interest, and I felt compelled to learn more.

I looked it up in the phone book. There was a listing for "crossfit," in all lowercase letters. It was a weekday in December 2001 when I dialed the number and heard a voice on the other end of the line. "Hello?"

The voice belonged to Greg Glassman, who I later learned was a personal trainer who had been kicked out of every gym he had worked in for his unconventional methods. Even more interesting was the fact that Glassman's original relocation, from Los Angeles to Santa Cruz, was to work with a team of deputies from the Santa Cruz County Sheriff's Office. Apparently, the training was too hard for the deputies, and he lost the contract. So he had gone out on his own and opened up his own gym.

"Come by tomorrow morning. Be here at 6." He gave me the address.

It was chilly the next morning, and as I drove along Research Park Drive, past a number of commercial facilities where you'd never think to find a gym, I thought, "I must have gotten this wrong." I pulled into a small parking lot next to a series of warehouse spaces, at an address that looked like a large storage unit, complete with a roll-up door.

Puzzled, I knocked twice. Greg Glassman answered the door with a smile and extended his hand. "You can call me Coach."

This is weird, I thought. The only people at the gym were me, Coach Glassman, and Mike Weaver, a black belt in jiu-jitsu who said he was there to do some extra training. Mike was the fiercest man I had ever seen in my life, with a razor-clean shaved head and thick cauliflower ear (or wrestler's ear). He would go on to become one of the first American black belts to win a jiu-jitsu tournament in Brazil. Legend had it that following the victory, he had to be escorted out of the country. One of Mike's great quotes was, "If you're doing CrossFit and competing in jiu-jitsu, then it's like you're cheating if your opponent is not."

The place didn't look at all like the gym we trained at during the academy. It was like something you'd see in a photo from a history book on old-school physical conditioning. Rather than the technology, machines, and mirrors I was accustomed to at a gym, this little place in an obscure part of Santa Cruz had items like medicine balls, barbells, a rope, and gymnastics rings hanging from the ceiling. Everything was clean and in order. The floor was pristine and there were Olympic weights and barbells neatly aligned and stacked. A large whiteboard hung on the wall.

Greg informed me that I would be working out against Mike. Against him? This statement just added more confusion to my situation. We were led up a flight of stairs to a shallow balcony that was home to two rowers.

We were told that we were going to start off with a 1,000-meter row. To which I thought, Big deal. We then went back down the steps, and I was introduced to my first kettlebell. Kettlebells were invented by Russian farmers in the 1700s as weights to measure crops. They were eventually introduced at local fairs for strongman competitions. The kettlebell looked about as old-school as a piece of exercise equipment could look, like a bowling ball-shaped hunk of iron with a handle forged onto it. Coach Glassman gave me one that weighed just 35 pounds. Mike had one that was probably about 53 pounds.

Thirty-five pounds. I thought, Are you kidding me? I wanted to protest and explain that I'd been trained at the Police Academy and had used much higher-level contraptions, like curl machines.

But I stopped myself, thinking: Be nice and be gracious. Don't judge it. But 35 pounds? Kind of a joke.

Then we were lead over to the pull-up bar. Pull-ups would apparently also be a part of this workout competition between Mike and me.

I had the plan: We would row 1,000 meters, then come down the steps and perform 21 of the kettlebell swings I had just been taught, then we would do 12 pull-ups.

"After you've completed one round," Coach informed me, "we'll think about a second."

My ego stirred again. Think? I must have forgotten to mention to him that before my training at the academy, I had played water polo for the University of California Santa Cruz.

We went back up the stairs and strapped ourselves into the rowing machines. Just before the workout started, Coach looked at me and said, "Kid, be careful walking down the stairs." Are you kidding me? Why on earth would I need to be careful on a simple staircase? In a booming voice, Coach announced the start of the workout: "3, 2, 1, go!" Mike and I ripped into the rowing machines.

This was my first time rowing, so I didn't know much about pacing, but I was a competitive person. The adrenaline of the "race" structure of the workout took hold.

I wanted to beat this guy. I wanted to beat this guy bad. My cop ego made this even more heated. I not only wanted to beat him in this 1,000-meter row, but I wanted to make it look like it didn't fatigue me in the least, that crushing him in this workout was a breeze.

That wasn't how it worked out. Mike bounded off the rower before I did, finishing the 1,000 meters and skipping down the stairs right to the kettlebell. I finally finished, having given everything I could muster. I didn't bound off the rowing machine like Mike. It was more of a crawl. I felt myself revisiting that drained, powerless feeling I had in my fight with the parolee. Everything was hazy. Once again it felt like I was desperately breathing through a straw.

As I made my way down the stairs, my legs felt rubbery, as if I had given a few pints of blood.

"Handrail! Handrail!" Coach cried out.

I straddled the kettlebell, wrecked and heaving for air. I had 21 swings to do. My scoffing at the 35-pound bell had come back to haunt me. My chest was still heaving and burning from the row. I could barely manage two or three swings at a time before I had to set the kettlebell on the ground.

After the 21st rep, I wobbled my way over to the pull-up bar. I wondered: Do I look as green as I feel? I was on the woozy edge of vomiting. I survived the pull-ups the same way I did the swings. Three, two, or one at a time. Mike had whizzed through them, using some sort of crazy gymnastics pull-up I later learned was called a kipping pull-up.

With regrettable form, I eked out the last of the 12 pull-ups. It was a freezing, foggy day in the coastal town of Santa Cruz, but I was burning up, ready to puke, pass out, or both. I crumbled into a heap at the bottom of the stairs, in the corner of the gym. Coach Glassman came over.

"Ready for that second round?"

I had been thoroughly humbled. A master of his work, Glassman never wasted energy trying to make the argument for his training philosophy or about why it was better than other programs. He just showed me by having me experience it.

For me, a cop determined to be better prepared for his job, I had found the physical training I was looking for.

In my pursuit of it, I took up the mentality of a white-belt in a first martial arts class. I accepted that I was a total beginner. I embraced Coach Glassman's model of high-intensity training using functional movements. A rapid series of results suggested I had made the right choice. In a short period of time, I made steep improvements at that little gym on Research Park Drive. Its value was apparent; I knew that this style of training would one day save my life.

The test came a few months later. I was on duty when the call came in: A wanted felon had been cornered on the second story of a condo. Three or four deputies formed a perimeter, while I was assigned to the entry team. I made entry and contacted the parolee in a bedroom on the second story of the condo. This guy had been in prison and it became clear that he wasn't going to get with the program. He jumped out the second-story window and hit the ground running full-tilt.

I ran down the stairs and began pursuit. The perimeter guys were chasing him as well. I began to pass them, swiftly gaining ground on the felon. I felt as though I was flying, with speed, stamina, and endurance to burn.

As I sprinted, the value of my new training vivid to everyone, including the felon, I burst out with words: "I've been training for this my whole life!"

I'm sure he heard me, but I'm still not sure whether he understood me or not. He definitely saw me charging at him. He threw his hands in the air and gave up.

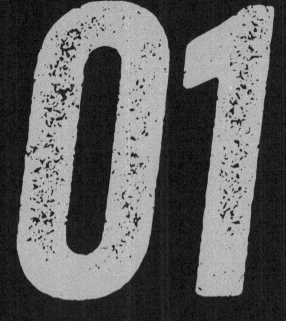

01

THE FIREBREATHER WAY

CROSSFIT WAS A MAJOR DISCOVERY for me, and I was all-in with this new way of physical training. I was impassioned and even began to gain a bit of notoriety as early videos of our workouts went viral on the Internet. Then there was the nickname "Firebreather." Early in my Cross-Fit training, I had just finished a brutal session, consisting of thrusters and pull-ups. Flat on my back, writhing in pain, throat burning, I looked over at my training partners, who were all experiencing the same discomfort. In a hoarse, scratchy voice, I said, "I feel like I'm breathing fire! It's like we are a bunch of firebreathers!" The name stuck, and it became a term of endearment and a great compliment to pay another athlete.

I was a Firebreather! At age 25, it seemed that I had reached the zenith of my athletic potential.

But I wasn't finished improving—I wanted to keep training and seeing gains. I came to realize that being a Firebreather meant more than just being physically developed. To continue to improve, it was key to embrace the totality of the training that went into integrating mind, body, and spirit.

Today I travel the country speaking to those working in the trenches of law enforcement. It's a complicated time. We live in an age of increasing chaos and confusion when it comes to serving and protecting people, when an act of domestic terrorism can be conducted by what amounts to a free agent, acting alone. It's also a time where trust of law enforcement is a serious issue for many communities. Having dedicated nearly two decades to serving in law enforcement and the military, I am passionate about this subject.

One response to this modern-day turmoil has been the acquisition of military-grade weapons and technologies by local police departments. The *New York Times* reported in 2014, "Police departments have received tens of thousands of machine guns; nearly 200,000 ammunition magazines; thousands of pieces of camouflage and night-vision equipment; and hundreds of silencers, armored cars and aircraft." Over the course of my career, technology has seemed to trump fitness in terms of importance.

I see this trend as the wrong way to go. My core message to the law-enforcement community is this: "The best weapon is you." When I say that, I'm talking about an officer who is fully tuned physically, mentally, and spiritually so that, whether on- or off-duty, he or she is capable of an optimal response to the chaos and unpredictability of any dangerous or unexpected situation.

That is a Firebreather state of mind and body. While the origin of the Firebreather nickname in my life focused on the physical, it was in my personal journey toward fulfilling my purpose—to be the absolute best I could be at my job, whether patrolling the streets as a cop or in a tactical battle with drug cartels as a DEA special agent—that the word became more robust for me.

My definition of Firebreather is two-pronged: (1) One who faces the triumphs and tribulations of great physical opposition with an indomitable spirit, and (2) An optimistic energy associated with the heart of an athlete.

Firebreather \fī(-ə)r-brē-thər\ (n)

1. One who faces the triumphs and tribulations of great physical opposition with an indomitable spirit.
2. An optimistic energy associated with the heart of an athlete.

I know from my own experience that following the Firebreather philosophy, which I will share and teach in the following chapters, is an optimal pathway to being an elite first responder, whether police officer, SWAT operator, soldier, or firefighter, so that when a violent situation erupts, he or she can be on top of it, performing at extraordinary levels of capacity in the face of the unknown and unknowable.

But hear this! Such a philosophy is *not* just for first responders. Everyone—regardless of background, age, work, and family—can adopt a similar form of training and discipline and realize the confidence, the self-reliance, and the power that comes with the optimization of body, mind, and spirit, all of which are integral to the Firebreather way.

The Firebreather Fitness program will empower you, regardless of background, status, or chosen pursuit, to live life with greater athletic capacity, mental prowess, and spiritual and emotional depth. And what's amazing is that you can step on that path today, right now, and in a matter of days and weeks begin to realize profound changes in productivity, physical performance, quality of life, an ability to stand out and lead, and develop a sense of calm, inner peace, and power.

Anyone can become a Firebreather if you are willing to do the work.

I believe you are ready to do the work. And I can show you the work that needs to be done. This book is your gateway.

Perhaps you are purely interested in being in the best *physical* shape of your life. You will certainly get there with the workouts in this program.

However, more is possible—much more. This program is intended as a game plan toward that *more*. Do you want to be able to respond to problems and challenging situations not with fear but with physical, mental, and emotional resiliency, along with strength, clear thinking, and resolve? To serve and be a model for others? To contribute more?

Being a Firebreather is not a destination—it's a state of mind. Commit yourself to the path. There's no doubt in my mind that if you perform the program consistently, you will reap long-term benefits, not just in those first 21 days, as some quick-start programs promise, but in the first year, and two years, and five years after that.

It might seem unusual to have a model of fitness that goes beyond the physical realm. After all, you've probably been drawn to a book like this from a desire to look and feel better—to burn off unwanted body fat, to build lean muscle tissue, to build (or rebuild) an athletic foundation. To be fit and to look fit. To unleash or restore your youth. Firebreather Fitness is all about those things. So then why am I so steadfast about building out the physical program in such a way that it also incorporates mental and spiritual dimensions?

Because I'm absolutely convinced, from my personal experience and that of thousands of people I've had an opportunity to teach and coach, that the route to not only achieving but *sustaining* peak fitness requires an integrated approach.

Let's face it: It's a long journey to the peak of your physical talent—toward being in the best physical condition of your life. It's a journey fraught with challenges, missteps, and setbacks. Blending mental and spiritual training into your physical program will give you the focus, resiliency, and discipline, plus an array of inner strengths to help you get the most out of every training session, each day, each week, month, and year, and over the course of years, in a fashion that is sustainable. It will help you stay the course and reach your potential.

As unusual as this integration of mind and spirit into body training may be to gym culture, there's nothing odd about it in the nearby dojo. For

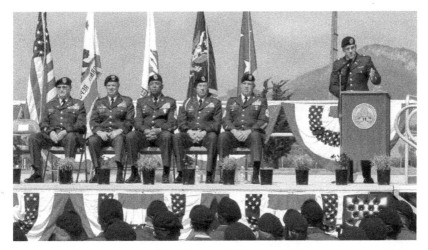

I was honored to give the 2006 graduation address at the US Army Officer Candidate School at Camp San Luis Obispo, California.

centuries, the best martial arts teachers have used a mix of movement and bodywork with meditation and mental-toughness training. There is no achieving great heights in martial arts without fully investing in the mental and spiritual dimensions of your training.

Firebreather Fitness fully embraces this approach to the work. The foundation that will emerge from this integration will provide you with a toolset so that when life trips you up, you will have an emotional resiliency and process to get you right back on track.

Believe me, I know from experience about being tripped up by life's curveballs.

A few years back, I experienced a series of emotionally charged incidents at the same time. My dog Baby, my companion for 12 years, unexpectedly died from cancer. Then my mom, whom I had not seen for over a year due to her service with the Peace Corps in Jordan, passed away from a brain tumor. My dad had passed away in 2000, which meant my three younger brothers and I were now without parents. The sudden illness and death of my mom launched my brothers and me into the uncertainty and financial hardship of dealing with hospital bills, burial planning, attorney fees, and our family estate. To complicate matters further, at the time of my mom's death, I was moving across California as I transitioned out of the Army and Drug Enforcement Administration (DEA) and into the private sector. As the world fell out from under me, my wife filed for divorce.

Somewhat ironically, this was during a time in my life when I was criss-crossing the country giving lectures on goal-setting and the value of positive self-talk. As someone who has served as a sheriff, a SWAT operator, a sniper, and a DEA agent in my primary career, and also as one of the original members of CrossFit who not only thrived in the program personally but taught thousands of prospective coaches in seminars around the country, I had developed exceptional performance capacities in all manner of stressful conditions, including those where lives were at stake.

But I was hit hard.

Many men and women, following a traumatic experience like divorce, spin out of control and turn to alcohol, drugs, overeating, anger, depression, and other unhealthy alternatives in an attempt to dilute their pain. Even with my background in elite-level law-enforcement training and long history in CrossFit, my personal situation severely tested my ability to navigate the kind of hard stuff that life can put on the table. I could feel a downward pull toward negativity and self-destruction.

For several months following the divorce, and really for the first time in my life, I felt utterly alone. Even after the loss of my beloved parents, I had never experienced such sadness, loneliness, and emotional stagnation. My days were spent in a fog, and I had a hard time sleeping at night. My distress stemmed from an inability to answer the question, "Where did I go wrong?" I had been a model of success in school, athletics, and business, and I had risen to the top in two simultaneous careers in the Army and Federal Law Enforcement. Yet I had failed where it mattered most.

I felt strongly that in order to focus on the lessons I needed to learn and to process the mistakes I'd made, I would need silence, seclusion, and living conditions that would deepen my connection to nature. I purchased an old Airstream motor home and leased a plot of land in the forest overlooking Aptos, California. With deer, rabbits, banana slugs, and birds as my new neighbors, I began an inward journey of self-reflection: my very own "vision quest" for knowledge, self-discovery, and the healing of a broken heart. In my isolation, I began to shed layers of ego and identity that had subconsciously driven my life in government service for nearly 14 years.

Although it was tempting, instead of falling off the path of my training into an unhealthy place of anger, self-medicating distraction, or emotional detachment, I chose to respond to the troubles and challenges with a Fire-breather mind-set. That meant rooting myself in the present moment with the conviction of facing and working my way through the distress toward better self-understanding, self-mastery, and eventually an inner peace.

Each morning, I awoke with the sunrise and meditated outside under redwood trees for hours at a time. I opened myself to listening to the inner wisdom in my heart, which had always been there, but had been dulled in the chaotic noise and fast pace of daily living.

One morning as I walked through the forest, I realized I had not uttered a word in more than five days. Silence embraced me, and I felt a profound peace. As I turned to walk back to my Airstream, a fawn appeared from behind a giant redwood tree and started to approach me. I stood very still, my arms extended at my sides with my palms open and visible to the deer, in a traditional martial artists nonthreatening posture. For what seemed an eternity, the deer and I held eye contact. This was the sign I had been look-ing for. I was at peace with myself and ready to move forward with my life.

I look back on that time with two thoughts in mind. The first is appre-ciation for those who were mentors for me. For it turns out I had never been alone at all—my life and training had been rich with teachers, coaches, mentors, and guides, who helped me to understand how valuable a holistic approach to fitness can be, and taught me how to not only embrace those difficult times that are inevitable to life but to learn from them. And the sec-ond: a compelling desire to pass along these lessons to anyone interested in a lifelong form of fitness development that is fun, powerful, and sustainable.

That's what this book is all about.

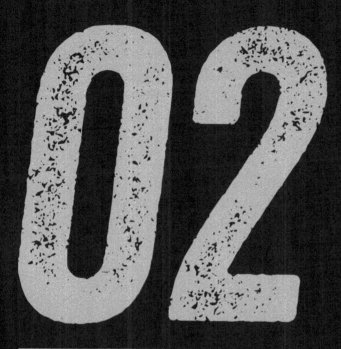

02

FIREBREATHING: A THREE-TIERED APPROACH

I RECALL A DRILL SERGEANT telling me and a group of young recruits at our induction into the US Army. "You'll all experience the Three Ds in my Army," he barked at us. "You'll get a divorce, your friends will die, and you'll deploy."

A similar sentiment was given to me during my training in the police academy. The instructor for family relations pulled a group of male recruits aside and said, "Just to warn you, cops have the highest divorce rate of any profession. Make sure you guys know a good attorney."

We all experience hardship and unwanted circumstances at different times in our lives; it's not just cops and soldiers. In fact, as I write this, Americans as a whole are dealing with a series of epidemics. Depression, drug addiction, and the obesity crisis are three problems that regularly make headlines. Over the past 15 years, the suicide rate has accelerated in the United States, up 30 percent for ages 35 to 64. For young Americans, suicide is the second-leading cause of death. We are living in a very stressful time that many of us are struggling to cope with.

I have a long history of training for stressful situations. I pursued my career in the police and military services with a warrior frame of mind—this would eventually evolve into what I call a Firebreather Mind-set. The idea was this: Times were stressful, and my life and the lives of others were on the line. Daily, I had to be at the top of my game in every respect—physically, mentally, spiritually.

Practically speaking, how did this mind-set affect my physical workouts? I pursued every workout as though it was the last workout I'd have before the fight of my life. My approach was that I needed to give every last ounce I could give, because it might be that final ounce that made a difference between triumph and coming up short and costing lives. My training focused on optimal performance, which meant pushing myself to train not just my body, but my mind and my spirit as well.

After all, the most important weapon a police officer has is a highly trained and fully integrated mind, body, and spirit, not his or her loaded gun. It goes way beyond muscles or a sophisticated piece of tactical gear. To think clearly and calmly, even in a heated situation, is imperative. To feel and project deep confidence is an amazingly powerful tool. A suspect picks up on that: Authentic confidence in a potentially violent situation will make the suspect think twice, and he or she will often back down and give up.

High-caliber mental capacities include things like coolness under pressure, mental and emotional resilience, and the ability to concentrate for long periods of time. There is no substitute in critical circumstances for the calm and confidence that come with good training.

To function at my highest level, I needed to build physical, mental, and spiritual fitness. Firebreather Fitness offers a long-term development of high performance and resilience. That kind of robust, holistic resilience is your best weapon in whatever challenges you face. It's also the firepower you need to get you to your goals, whatever they may be.

THE FIREBREATHER DIFFERENCE

The Firebreather Fitness program offers three levels (beginner, intermediate, and advanced) as well as scaling options for the movements. This allows the training to become accessible to anyone willing to do the work, no matter what his or her starting point. The Firebreather path is truly open to all.

By embracing a high-intensity/low-volume exercise program with constantly varying functional movements, I have been able to produce high-level health and fitness gains for 16 years and counting. You can too. Not only that, you will lay a foundation for any and every sport imaginable.

But if physical training is all that Firebreather Fitness is about, it wouldn't be much different from 100 other workout programs. A basic physical fitness program is better than nothing, certainly, but by itself, it may fail to adequately prepare a person for the hectic, stressful lifestyle that the age of high technology has helped usher in.

Firebreather Fitness goes beyond merely a physical program. It offers a path toward the preparation necessary not only to meet daily demands but also to improve quality of life, to reconnect with the energy and power of nature, and to develop mental and spiritual disciplines that offer tools to influence the perspective by which we see the world.

Unfortunately, conventional fitness is limited in dimension, purpose, and use. Large commercial gyms are built on a business model that doesn't really have your fitness in mind. To such places, the ideal gym member is one who signs up, swipes a credit card and signs a contract, then never shows up again. Gyms that offer memberships as low as $20 or $10 per month are the most obvious examples of this model.

Clients who do show up often do so without a significant purpose or intent in their training. This has been talked about a lot in recent years, with the rise of the CrossFit model a strong counterpoint. Unlike traditional gym training, CrossFit training is a community-based conditioning program based on constantly varying functional movements performed at high intensity. It uses strict definitions and is purpose-based, focused on building an all-around athletic foundation.

But even great physical workouts like those are often missed opportunities to integrate that physical training with mental and spiritual training. There is a tendency to compartmentalize training, putting the training of the body, the training of the mind, and the forging of the spirit into different categories, as if they are separate. In fact, these all must be interconnected to actualize potential.

In Firebreather Fitness, the physical, mental, and spiritual exercises are woven into a single program.

1 BODY

People go to the gym with myriad objectives. Losing weight is the most common. Some want to build a certain kind of body, maybe to imitate what they've seen on magazine covers, and are drawn to bodybuilding programs. Others want a fitness program to support their sport, be it running, biking, surfing, skiing, or what have you. Others want to have more energy, or aspire to look and feel younger. What's the right approach?

Firebreather Fitness brings simplicity to this often-confusing subject. Because here's the secret about physical training: The single best way to accomplish any and all of these goals is the same: a core strength and conditioning program that relies on compound, functional movements and focuses on performance.

I'm in my 30s, as strong and lean as I was 10 years ago, and I'm often asked how I was able to build the body I have. My answer is always the same: I didn't target a specific body type. Instead, I focused on performance, and the body I have is a by-product of the work and capacity I have achieved. I've focused solely on performance, and my form and physique are a direct causation of that effort. Make performance gains your focus, and your body will naturally take care of the rest.

When you chase performance, your body will develop in alignment with the body you were meant to have. A natural, healthy, mobile, toned, and resilient physical expression of your physique is a by-product of adherence to the Firebreather program.

Focusing on performance means following a program where gains can be clearly measured. For example, in week four, you can do five pull-ups. In week eight, you are able to do eight pull-ups. In Firebreather Fitness, we measure progress with concrete, measurable data points, from how fast you can run 2 miles to personal time records with various workouts, to the range of motion you have in performing a yoga routine, to your positive mind-set and clear definition of your life purpose.

To make the most gains, we target functional, compound movements; eat real, healthy foods; and let nature take care of the rest. Whether your fitness goals are building muscle, increasing energy, or health and wellness, all of these can result from using simple exercises. You don't need fancy equipment or a pricey gym to carry out and enjoy a lifetime's worth of personal improvement through my program. You will be amazed at how much can be accomplished on a patch of grass simply using your body, the Earth's gravity, and a mix of functional exercises. You don't need three hours a day, either. Your desired results can be accomplished in only 20 minutes a day when you mix an energized sense of intention with a purposeful set of functional exercises.

Do you need to lift weights? By all means, I encourage you to add resistance training with weights to your program, but I also highly endorse a tree branch, a park bench, and a jump rope—all potentially transformative exercise tools when put to use correctly and consistently. If you want to build your own garage gym, that will help you add even more enjoyment and variety into your program. But if you just have a local park or a small, carpeted area to work with, you can do wonders with the principles in this book.

2 MIND

CrossFit founder Greg Glassman offered me this profound insight: "The greatest adaptation to CrossFit takes place between the ears."

His point was that getting into top physical condition—both in terms of optimal body type and optimal performance—has a lot to do with the right mental toolset. This insight is the foundation for why I believe integrating mental training into your fitness program is essential. I would add to Coach's words this: A *sustainable and integrated fitness program* happens between the ears!

Consider how many people start fitness programs but never really get into them or see any results. Or make the all-too-common mistake of going at it too hard and too fast in the beginning and then burning out.

Something I've seen often in my own gym is the super-motivated beginner who comes in on Day One wearing new workout clothes, expensive new shoes, and an eager expression. They come in charged up but then vanish within a few weeks, never to be seen again.

When I encounter athletes who fit this description, my strategy is always to slow things down and to help them set incremental goals that they can focus on in the first few months of training. I encourage them to pace themselves through a process that will help them become comfortable with a type of discomfort that will make for improvements. I know that if they don't do that, they are in danger of burning through all of that fantastic enthusiasm like a rocket burning through most of its fuel prior to takeoff.

A sustainable and integrated fitness program happens between the ears!

If you've struggled with connecting to an exercise program that you can sustain over a long period of time, then I urge you to accompany your physical workouts with a combination of mind-set tools. These tools include things such as setting smart goals, supporting those goals with the right self-talk language, and training your mind in the art of positive self-expectation.

The Firebreather Fitness 21-day plans supplement the physical workouts with these mental tools. By integrating mental training into your physical training program, you will unleash a type of power and energy that will develop the results you are looking for, both in the near- and far terms. Don't be surprised to find this power spilling over into every other area in your life, as well.

3 SPIRIT

Discussing spiritual strength during a conversation about fitness may seem out of sync to some, but when it comes to athleticism and supreme fitness, spirit is a core subject. As I'll discuss in a later section of the book, spirit is woven throughout the entire Firebreather Fitness program.

Spirit energizes the purpose we bring to our training and to our lives. It is your energy source when training gets uncomfortable and hard, for example, in the final miles of a marathon or two-thirds of the way through an epic workout. Spirit is what allows you to push harder and farther into extreme challenge and accomplishments.

Some sports, such as surfing, skiing, ultrarunning, and hiking, have a spiritual element built in to them, allowing a deep connection with nature. Traditional martial artists practitioners put the spirit of the discipline first when it comes to their training.

In the Native American warrior tradition, the development of spirit was critical in the maturation of a young warrior. "The great spirit that moves through all living things" was earnestly sought by the warrior. Discovering and honoring this great spirit that is within you, and everyone else, is a key component to the Firebreather Fitness program.

The bottom line? Living up to all of our potential means engaging and developing *all* that we are, our spiritual selves alongside our physical selves.

The Firebreather Fitness program offers a focused plan to train body, mind, and spirit in short, daily episodes. We will start in the physical realm, with an overview of the fundamental movements used in the program.

BODY

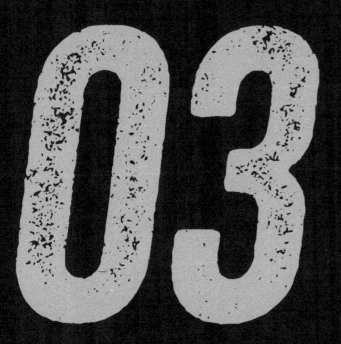

03

FOUNDATIONAL MOVEMENTS

THE EXERCISES IN THE FIREBREATHER PLAN are grounded in functional, compound movements that activate groups of muscles to work together in peak fashion. When you perform a real-life athletic movement you never use just a single muscle to do it. Rather, these movements are combinations of muscles being fired in complementary patterns. In other words, compound movements are how we function as human beings to get physical work done. They are how we lift furniture on moving day or play a sport: lifting, jumping, throwing, pulling, pushing, running.

This chapter highlights the movements I consider the most important. Some are also building blocks toward more demanding movements. A push-up, for instance, is a stepping stone toward the more athletically demanding handstand push-up. The kinetic chain of energy used to snap a kettlebell upward into a swing helps ingrain a complicated sequence of motor recruitment patterns that will help you clean and jerk hundreds of pounds of weight off the floor and up over your head in Olympic lifting.

Give these descriptions a thorough read, in order to get the technique down. All exercises, even the simplest ones, such as a push-up or pull-up, are most beneficial when you take steps to do them correctly. As you begin the Firebreather Fitness 21-day plan, you will likely find yourself returning to this chapter again and again as you work toward mastering these moves. I promise that after a few weeks of experiencing how they get your heart pumping and develop your body and fitness in complete ways, you'll be a believer.

THE FOUR PATTERNS

Several years ago, I realized that the essential movement patterns that I needed to train could be reduced to four categories of movement: open, close, push, pull. I discovered that as long as I touched base with these patterns consistently, I was ready for action. The foundational movements in this book represent one or more of these four basic patterns.

OPEN

"Open" refers to the ability of the ankle, knee, and hip to reach full extension—also known as triple extension. The majority of the skills we employ in the Firebreather plans have either an open quality to them in the context of triple extension, or a static contraction through these same joints. For example, in a squat, you reach triple extension and open the body, whereas in a push-up, you maintain a static contraction through the same joints. The ankle, knee, and hip remain isometrically in extension, while the upper body moves from a retracted to an extended position through the push-up.

CLOSE

To "close" the body refers to a movement that dynamically shortens the line of axis from the chest to the hip. Two examples are the sit-up and the toes to bar progression. The body is closing, or folding, at the hip, under tension. Notice that from the top of the squat to the bottom position, there is also a closing element. However, I advocate choosing a specific range of motion that really accentuates the closing nature of the skill.

PUSH

To "push" with the body refers to any skill that extends an object away from the center of the body's mass. For example, a push-up moves the body away from the floor at the moment of extension through the elbow, shoulder, and chest. A jerk or press moves a barbell away from the center of mass with an extension of the hip and arms, and the acceleration of weight overhead. Note that in some pushing movements, as in the push press, the hip and knee are involved, adding both a pushing and opening quality.

PULL

To "pull" with the body refers to your ability to bring an object closer to your center of mass. For example, in a pull-up, from extension, you pull your body closer to the bar.

MANY TIMES, the compound multi-joint exercises you are asked to do in the Firebreather Fitness program blend various components of the open, close, push, and pull together. This is the beauty of the program, as it lends itself to quick gains in fitness.

PREPARING FOR THE UNKNOWN

My concept of the open, close, push, and pull movements was born out of necessity and a compelling desire to be ready for the "unknown and unknowable" daily workout that Coach Glassman would prescribe to the athletes training under his care at 6:00 a.m. In the early days of my CrossFit training, there was no website, and every morning when I arrived at the gym, I had to prepare myself mentally and physically for whatever Coach wrote on the whiteboard.

At first, warming up and preparing for an unknown task—one that would be performed in an extremely competitive environment—was overwhelming. However, one morning something struck me about the nature of the compound, multi-joint movements that always made up the workouts Coach created. Regardless of the programming, the weight, the repetition scheme, or the order of events, I could count on the workout to ask of my body four general ranges of motion: extending at the ankle, knee, and hip (the open movement category); closing at the axis of the hip (the close movement category); pulling my body up the rope, onto the rings, or onto the pull-up bar (the pull movement category); or pushing an object away from my center of mass (the push movement category).

I always included in my warm-up the following exercises, each performed for 10 repetitions:

Overhead squat (the supreme open movement)

Toes-to-bar (a favorite close movement)

Handstand push-up (a powerful skill that focuses solely on upper-body pushing power and strength)

Pull-up (a pull movement that is a combination of strict and kipping, with a variety of grip choices to mix things up)

Warming up my open, close, push, and pull movement patterns helped jump-start my confidence so that I was ready, both physically and mentally, to attack any and all of the challenging workouts Coach Glassman wrote on the whiteboard.

BODY-WEIGHT BASICS

There are no excuses when it comes to hopping onto the path of optimal conditioning. You don't need a gym membership or elliptical trainer or a pair of expensive running shoes. You can start with some space on the floor or the ground, or a trip to a playground to use a bar for pull-ups.

Any doubt about the effectiveness of body-weight exercises can be dismissed by watching the feats and physiques of good gymnasts. Gymnastics is a primal language of athletics and sport and where it all begins.

The exercises on the following pages are a great place to start. Once you have mastered the basic techniques, try scaling up to increase strength and performance.

AIR SQUAT

>> The air squat is foundational not only to being a good athlete but also to being a functional human being. If you were to use only one exercise in your life, I'd make a strong argument for choosing the air squat. It is the starting point for the **open** category of skills.

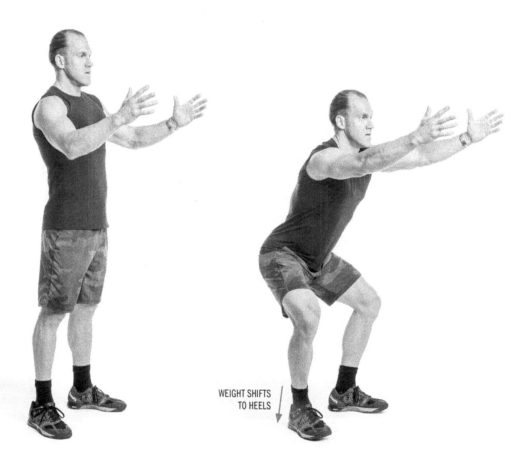

WEIGHT SHIFTS
TO HEELS

1 Feet are between hip- and shoulder-width apart, with toes slightly canted out, weight firmly rooted in heels. Arms are up in an athletic-ready position. Lower body is extended at ankle, knee, and hip.

2 Keeping gaze neutral to ensure a single line of action from hip to crown of head, begin to push butt back and down. The key word is "push."

The squat is not a gravity-assisted exercise; rather, the descent is an active and fully engaged motion. As hip descends, continue to lift arms farther away from butt. The length of the arms helps keep chest up.

3 Push butt back and down. As butt moves backward, focus on keeping chest up, and lift your arms, which keeps chest up.

POINTS OF PERFORMANCE

In the early days of my CrossFit training, Coach Glassman told me, "Greg, you've got to master the squat, because the squat is the ultimate hip-extension movement." When I asked Coach to explain the significance of the hip extension, he said, "Because powerful and controlled hip extension is a requirement of elite human performance." This was a real awakening for me!

SCALING

A tough aspect of the air squat for beginners is that they might have some mobility restriction in the back, hip, or ankles. Begin by focusing on quality, sinking into a deep squat and holding it as long as you can. You may brace yourself by holding a beam, but work toward longer and longer squat holds where you are doing the work yourself.

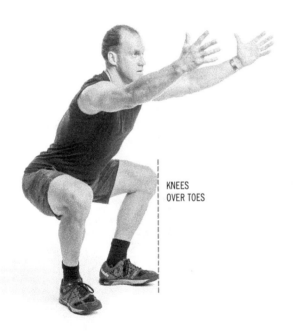

KNEES
OVER TOES

4 The bottom position brings the crease of the hip below the knee. Knees track over the feet, and weight remains in the heels. Maintain lumbar curve throughout the entire movement.

5 With a strong contraction of the legs, drive through heels to return to top position. Shoulders and hips rise at the same rate and arms return to the start position.

LUNGE

One of my favorite lower-body conditioning skills, the lunge helps build strength as well as balance, coordination, timing, and power. The lunge is in the **open** category of skills.

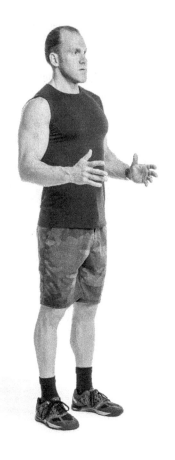

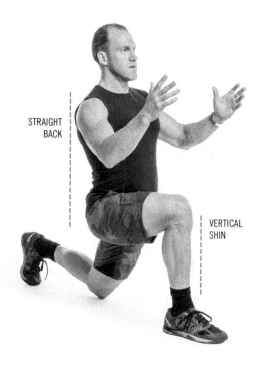

STRAIGHT
BACK

VERTICAL
SHIN

1 From a standing position, step forward with the right foot. Place foot directly in front of you.

2 Keeping upper body upright, gently kiss left knee to the ground. Contact should be light and gentle. Note vertical shin angle of right leg.

3 Press off ground with right leg, and in one fluid motion return to standing.

SCALING

There are a variety of ways to modify and scale the lunge. The first step is to reduce the range of motion and come into a "quarter lunge." As strength and mobility increases, the depth of the rear leg will also increase, ultimately achieving full range of motion.

A great mental-toughness challenge is the 400-meter walking lunge. Walk forward for 400 meters, using the lunge skill taught above. Rest in the top standing position between steps, or step forward into the next repetition.

An advanced variation is the weighted lunge. Hold weights or kettlebells, which builds incredible grip strength, in addition to leg strength.

BOX JUMP

>> The box jump is a tremendous skill that develops explosive hip-opening capacity, power, coordination, and speed. This skill is in the **open** category. For women, I recommend starting with a 16-inch box and progressing to a 20-inch box. For men, begin with a 20-inch box and progress to a 24-inch box. The advanced, long-term goal is a 24-inch box for women and 30-inch box for men.

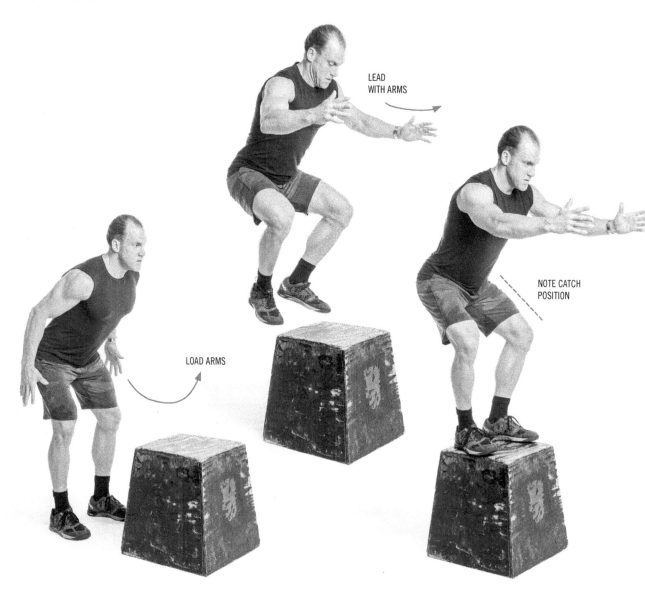

LEAD WITH ARMS

LOAD ARMS

NOTE CATCH POSITION

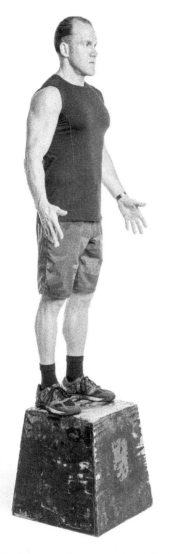

POINTS OF PERFORMANCE

The box jump is a hip-extension exercise, not a leg-extension exercise. This skill significantly increases your ability to open the hip with explosive speed and power. Therefore, rather than squatting deeply in front of the box, slightly bend forward and load your arms. At most, the legs bend a few inches.

SCALING

For an added challenge, try plyometric box jumps. Start on top of the box, jump down to the floor, and use the stretch reflex of your calves to spring back onto the box. It's best to learn this skill with a shorter box than you normally train with, and gradually increase the height of the box.

Another scaling option is to step onto the box, rather than jump. When stepping, ensure you extend the working leg entirely before the other foot touches the box. In this manner, you allow one leg to lift the body at a time. This is also a great way to isolate one leg at a time, and helps to develop strength for the single-leg squat.

1 Start by standing approximately six inches from the box with feet set under hips. Bend slightly forward and load the arms.

2 Lead with the arms. Let arms and hands accelerate the rest of your body onto the box.

3 Land evenly on the box and catch yourself as high as possible. A common fault is to land on the box in the bottom of a squat.

4 Jump or step directly down, resetting to the jump position.

SINGLE-LEG SQUAT

>> The single-leg squat (aka "the pistol") develops leg strength, balance, agility, coordination, and incredible abdominal strength. Think of this skill as core development, as opposed to just leg strength. This skill is in the **open** category of skills.

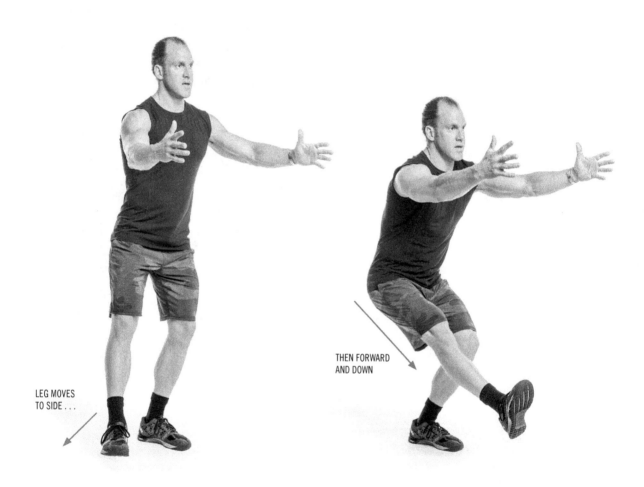

LEG MOVES
TO SIDE . . .

THEN FORWARD
AND DOWN

1 From a traditional squat position, bring all weight into the support foot/squatting leg. Contract midsection and inhale through nose.

2 As hips press back and down, extend non-support leg out to the side and then, as you squat, extend leg forward.

3 At the bottom position, hip is below squatting leg and chest is up. Arms are extended forward, with opposing hand reaching slightly toward extended foot. This action of cross-body rotation helps align the hips and shoulders, and keeps spine in alignment.

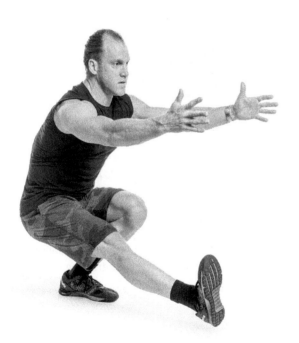

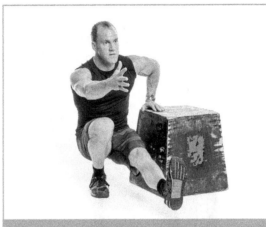

SCALING

To scale the single-leg squat, one great option is to use a box: A box can help you balance and also can be used as leverage. Ensure that you keep your body perfectly aligned if using a box for assistance. A common fault is to collapse toward the box. Place the box aside the extended leg, and use it during any "sticky" point of the repetition. As soon as the leg can take over, reduce or remove the assistance of the arm.

4 To return to the top position, contract midsection. Press through heel as extended leg returns through the same range of motion as the descent. A slight exhalation making a "hissing sound" to increase inner-abdominal pressure can help the ascent.

TOES-TO-BAR PROGRESSION

>> Toes-to-bar, a **close** movement, is an unbeatable core-strength/trunk-strength exercise. A key part of learning the skill is understanding the progression between the knee raise, knees-to-elbow, and toes-to-bar. I encourage practicing and learning the skills in this order, which will increase your overall development and midline strength.

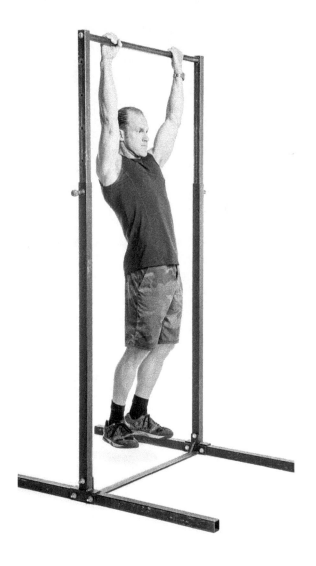

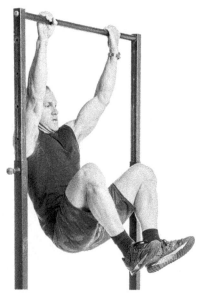

KNEE RAISE

1 Begin in full extension with arms just outside shoulders, gripping bar in a reverse grip. Maintain an active shoulder position; you are not in a deadman's hang (see page 42) but rather actively pulling scapula back and down, and contracting through the side body.

2 Contract arms and upper back, and raise knees above midline, or belly button.

3 Bring feet back down through the same line of action, being careful to not let the feet swing behind you.

Continue to practice and gain proficiency with this skill, gradually increasing the height of the knee raise, with a goal of touching your knees to your elbows.

SCALING

In this progression, each exercise builds your strength to progress to the next. Use knee raise as a stepping stone to knees-to-elbow, building up to toes-to-bar.

POINTS OF PERFORMANCE

Following the toes-to-bar, the key is developing consecutive repetitions, and this can be achieved by bringing the feet back to the starting position along the same line of action as the ascent. A common fault is "casting" the toes straight out, rather than down. Returning the feet along a nearly straight line of action to the start position ensures fast, consecutive repetitions without unnecessary back swing of the legs.

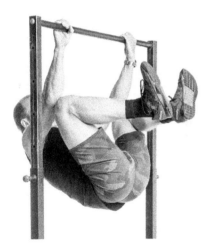

KNEES-TO-ELBOW

1 Knees-to-elbow continues the line of action from knee raise—instead of stopping at midline, continue to lift knees until they contact the elbow. A common fault is only touching knees to triceps. The greatest contraction through the midline occurs when you curl into a ball and make knee-to-elbow contact.

2 Bring feet back down through the same line of action, being careful to not let feet swing behind you.

Continue to practice and gain proficiency with this skill, preparing for a goal of touching your toes to the bar.

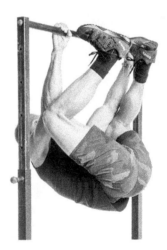

TOES-TO-BAR

1 Contract arms and upper back, curling at the waist, and bringing toes to touch the bar. Note body position at the top of the skill is compact, with arms slightly bent, and knees move to the outside of the elbows.

2 Bring feet back down through the same line of action, being careful to not let the feet swing behind you.

PUSH-UP

>> Push-ups involve a classic push movement. They are a mainstay in the training of military personnel, and for good reason: They can be performed anytime, anywhere, and they are effective. It's not just a chest exercise; push-ups require core and trunk strength, and work muscles throughout the entire body. The push-up is in the **push** category of fitness skills.

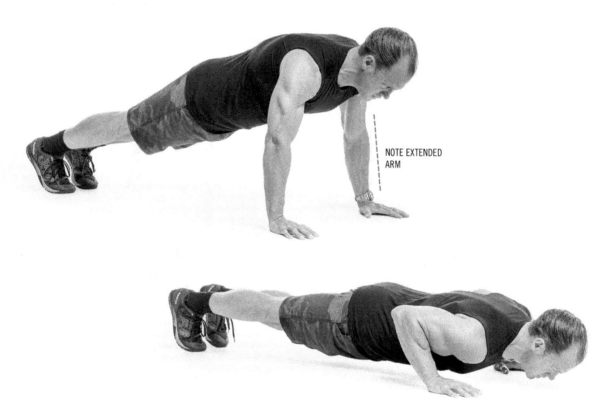

NOTE EXTENDED ARM

1 Begin in plank position, with hands stacked directly underneath shoulders. The entire body becomes a single unit with a strong contraction through the midsection. Gaze is down, allowing for proper alignment along the spine. Scapula are in a retracted position, allowing for engagement in the large muscles of the back during the skill.

2 Maintaining a straight line of action from heels of your feet to the crown of your head, pull down to the bottom position. The descent to the bottom position is active, not gravity assisted. In the bottom position, chest hovers approximately one inch off the ground.

POINTS OF PERFORMANCE

Focus on your midline and "core" for the duration of the movement. Although most people think of the push-up as an upper-body builder, which it is, there is also ample opportunity to develop incredible midline strength. Try to imagine your body as a single integrated unit from heels to hands during each repetition.

SCALING

Knee push-ups are not ideal because they reduce the trunk-strengthening value of the push-up. The best scaling option is to do the best quality push-ups you can muster. Just do fewer. Also, holding a plank for long periods of time is a great way to build the infrastructure strength for push-ups. Start with 20-second plank holds and work up to 1 minute or longer. Be sure to hold perfect form throughout: Letting your alignment break and your belly sag near the floor does more harm than good.

3 Contracting arms, back, and chest, press through the floor to return to the top position. Do the full push-up, not a half or quarter push-up. The full range of motion ensures your arms are completely extended, while your shoulder blades are simultaneously retracted.

DIP

>> The dip, often regarded as an upper-body squat by coaches, is a vital skill in any strength and conditioning program. It can be performed on a dip bar or on the rings for added challenge. The dip is in the **push** category of skills.

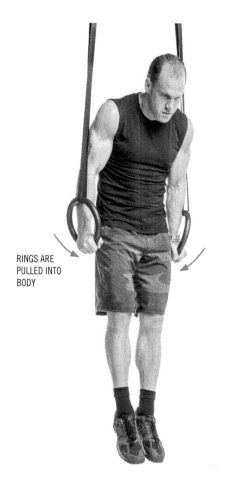

RINGS ARE
PULLED INTO
BODY

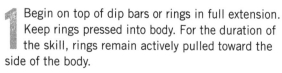

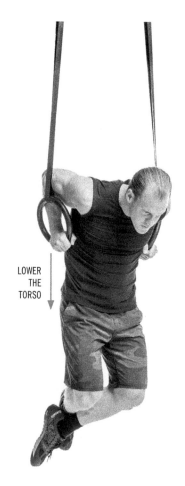

LOWER
THE
TORSO

1 Begin on top of dip bars or rings in full extension. Keep rings pressed into body. For the duration of the skill, rings remain actively pulled toward the side of the body.

2 Lower hip and torso in a straight line of action by bending the elbows. A common fault is to simply bend at the waist, without moving the hips.

3 As elbows rise above shoulders and hips descend, allow chest to naturally come forward, no greater than a 45-degree angle. Note that rings are touching chest.

4 With a strong contraction of arms, shoulders, and chest, press back along the same line of action to return to full extension.

POINTS OF PERFORMANCE

The ring dip adds considerable challenge to the stability of the bar dip. This is due to the inherent instability of the ring. A great way to achieve the strength necessary for the rings is to first achieve capacity with the bar dip. Think of two bar dips as equal to one ring dip.

SCALING

If you are struggling with the dip, the best way to build strength for this skill is push-ups. With ring dips, you can also thread a resistance band through the rings and then hook the band under a foot.

HANDSTAND PUSH-UP

Handstand push-ups are a powerful strengthener; one is equal to about 10 push-ups from the floor. Shoulder strength developed though the handstand push-up is world-class. The handstand push-up is in the **push** category of skills.

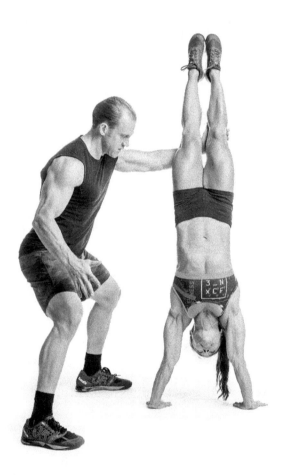

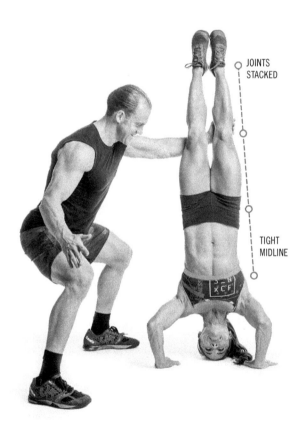

JOINTS STACKED

TIGHT MIDLINE

1 Stand alongside a training partner with hands set just outside shoulders and fingers spread for balance.

2 In a controlled, graceful manner, kick up one foot at a time, with assistance from the partner, as necessary.

3 Maintain a solid midline position, keeping shoulders over hands. Hips are stacked over shoulders, and legs are in full extension. Every muscle in the body is engaged.

4 Lower head to the ground between hands, then extend arms, and return to start position.

POINTS OF PERFORMANCE

Perform this skill solo by using the support of a wall instead of a partner to hold your feet.

SCALING

To work your way up to a handstand push-up, the first step is a 1:00 handstand hold (follow only steps 1 to 3). Then work the eccentric phase of the skill, slowly lowering head to floor, before returning feet to the floor. Kick feet back up, returning to top position, and repeat for desired number of repetitions. A great tempo for the descent in this drill is 10 seconds.

Annie Sakamoto, my longtime friend and training partner, was my first choice as a model to help demonstrate the exercises in the Firebreather Fitness program. She exemplifies all the qualities of a Firebreather, from her commitment to virtuosity to her kindness and spirit of goodwill. Annie is a great testimony to the power of commitment, hard work, personal belief, and a strong sense of purpose.

RING ROW

The ring row is a fantastic upper-body strength and conditioning exercise, and one that will quickly yield the strength required for the strict pull-up. It is a **pull** skill that also has an element of static contraction (or: open) through the midsection.

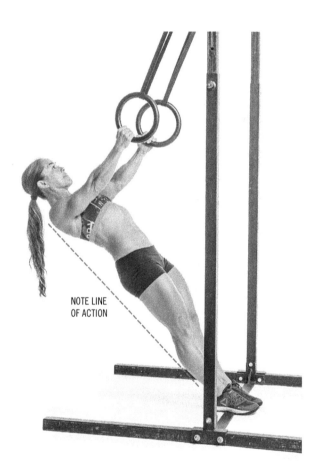

NOTE LINE
OF ACTION

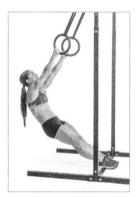

Note that in the incorrect position Annie has lost her midline stability, and her upper back has rounded out.

1 Set rings at shoulder level. Standing with feet directly under rings, grip rings, and lean backward.

2 Maintain an active shoulder position by retracting the scapula—squeezing the shoulder blades as if you were trying to hold a grapefruit onto your upper spine. The line of action from feet to shoulder should be a straight line.

POINTS OF PERFORMANCE

When done correctly, the ring row powerfully develops your midline strength and stability, as well as upper-body strength.

SCALING

To scale down, step backward, away from the center point of the rings. This decreases the distance your body travels during the skill. To scale up, step forward. For the ultimate challenge, elevate feet onto a box in front of you.

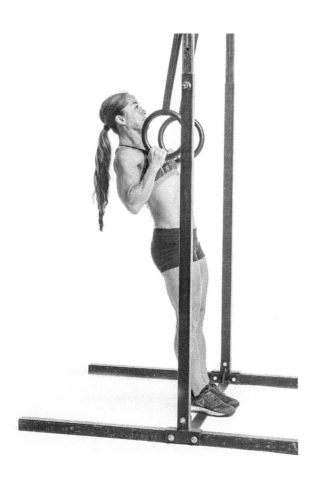

3 Keeping body in a single plane, contract arms and upper back, and pull yourself up to rings. Finishing position is touching the rings to shoulders.

PULL-UP

A classic **pull** movement, the pull-up is simple yet exceptionally effective and exercises muscles throughout the body.

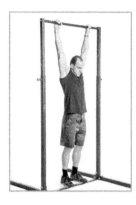

Note that in the "dead hang" version I have lost all contraction through my shoulder and back. This is a very disadvantageous starting position. Correct start position has the shoulders rotated back and down, and a strong contraction through the entire back.

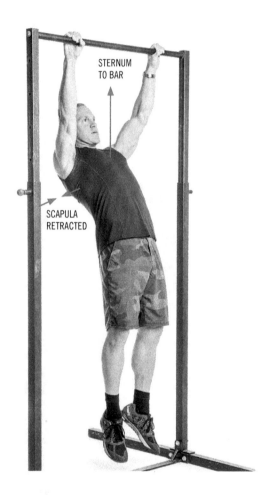

STERNUM TO BAR

SCAPULA RETRACTED

GRIPS

CHIN-UP

PULL-UP

REVERSE GRIP

There are several types of grips that you can use for any bar-type movement, whether it's a pull-up, toe-to-bar, or knee-to-elbow. A traditional "chin-up" grip has palms facing away from you. The "pull-up" grip has palms facing you, and the "reverse grip" has an alternate grip, similar to what you will see on the deadlift technique. Coach Glassman once told me, "You want to get to a point where using any grip with any object—whether bar, tree branch, or stairwell railing—you can grab and pull yourself up."

1 From an overhand position on the pull-up bar, with thumb wrapped around the bar, begin with a strong retraction of the scapula. This action brings the torso closer to the bar, ensures a strong shoulder position, and allows for greater engagement in the muscles of the back. Note: As the scapula retracts, the angle of the torso in relation to the bar changes. Your sternum will point to the bar, opening the chest and preparing the back to pull.

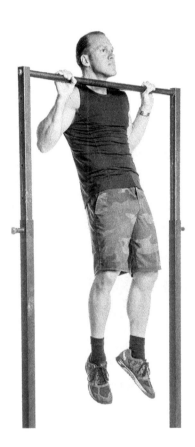

POINTS OF PERFORMANCE

The key for the strict pull-up is to focus on retracting the scapula, drawing the shoulder blades together. Note the different starting positions in the "dead hang" and the "active hang." In the active position, I have created the optimum pulling position, ensuring the large muscles in my back are involved in the pull-up, rather than just relying on my arms. This principle alone has helped hundreds of law-enforcement officers on their SWAT assessment test.

SCALING

To scale down, use assistance from a box or resistance band to achieve the top position. Once at the top, lower to bottom position over a 10-second count. From the bottom, immediately return to the top with assistance from the band, jumping from a box, or having a partner give you a boost. Repeat the slow, controlled descent.

To scale up, add a weight belt that holds a weight (usually a kettlebell), or hold a dumbbell between crossed legs.

Ring rows are another fantastic way to achieve strength in the pull-up. Using them, you can modify the level of difficulty. (See ring row, page 40.)

2 Pulling from back and arms, direct sternum toward the bar. Maintain this angle of approach, finally bringing chin over the bar once the proper height has been established. Maintaining the angle of the chest until the last moment ensures that you engage through the back for the duration of the skill.

3 Lower through a straight line of action to the start position. Be sure to "put the brakes on" and don't allow yourself to return to a dead-hang position.

JUMP ROPE

>> Jumping rope is an excellent **conditioning** and coordination skill that improves timing, accuracy, coordination, and agility. Double unders, where the rope passes beneath you twice in one jump, take practice, but with patience, you will master them. You might want to practice proper jumping position without a rope first.

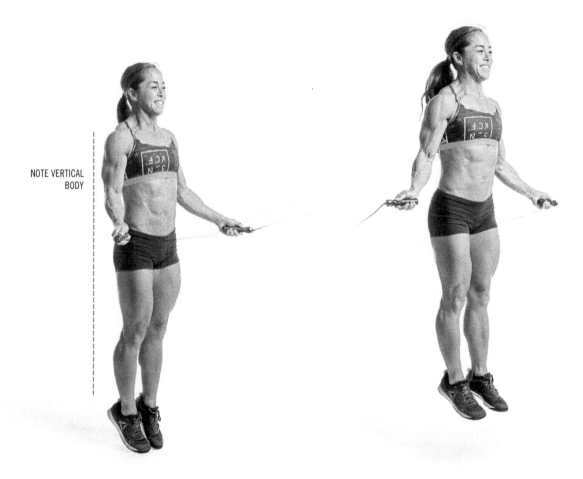

NOTE VERTICAL BODY

1 Begin to spin the rope, keeping hands close to sides and focusing on a speedy rotation of wrist, not elbow or shoulder.

2 Jump lightly off the balls of your feet. Your heels should never touch the ground. A common fault is the donkey kick, in which you contract the hamstrings and bring the heels backward.

POINTS OF PERFORMANCE

To learn double unders, I set a timer for 5:00 and simply practiced. I allowed myself to trip, get stuck, and flail around. I knew I just needed time with the rope, and that with practice, I would succeed. Set microgoals, starting with a goal of 5 consecutive double unders, and increasing to 10, with a long-term goal of 100. There is a tendency to tense up doing this skill. Remember to relax, breathe deeply and evenly, and remain in place as you jump lightly off the ground. Finally, if necessary, start your double unders with just one single. It can be hard on the timing to transition from multiple single jumps to double unders, so give yourself one single only in order to get rope speed, then immediately transition to a double under.

Note: The difference between a single jump and a double under is the speed of the rope's rotation, not the height of the jump. A common fault is jumping too high, which leads to quick muscle fatigue.

BURPEE

The burpee, which combines the squat and the push-up, builds strength, power, and mobility. It's a terrific conditioning movement. It should be treated as a highly technical skill, as opposed to simply flopping onto the ground and standing back up. Well-executed transitions in the burpee develop speed, agility, coordination, and balance. The burpee draws from both the **open** and **push** categories.

1 Begin in an upright, athletic-ready position. The initial line of action is nearly identical to a squat. Push butt back and down, while lifting arms and chest.

2 As you approach the bottom of the squat, kick feet backward while placing hands on ground. At beginning levels, place hands on ground first, then jump or step feet back. At advanced levels, hands and feet touch at the same moment, following a period of airborne suspension.

3 Once in plank position, transition through a controlled push-up. Return to top position of plank.

4 With a strong contraction of the midsection, tuck knees to chest while lifting chest and arms. Return to bottom position of squat. Similar to transition from squat to plank, in the return from plank to squat, there is a moment of airborne suspension and weightlessness that is contrasted with the aggressive and controlled reset at the bottom of the squat.

5 Driving explosively through the heels, extend legs, open hip, and jump off the ground. The height of the jump can vary: at least jump high enough to allow hands to clap overhead while feet are off the ground.

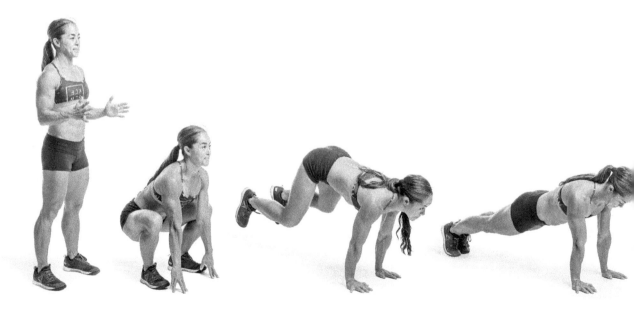

POINTS OF PERFORMANCE

Focus on a straight body position in the plank and push-up positions. For safety of the low back, and development of midline stability and strength, it is important to move the body as a single unit during the plank and push-up phases. A common fault is snaking up, which divides your lower and upper body in half and negates the potential to develop real strength through the midsection.

Jump straight up. Imagine you're diving into a swimming pool, and your goal is to score a perfect 10 with no splash. To accomplish this, you must open at the hip and engage the erector muscles in the low back to allow you to stack joints all the way from your fingertips, through your elbows, shoulders, spine, hip, knees, and ankles. To keep your jump honest, jump to an object set 6 inches above your fully extended arm.

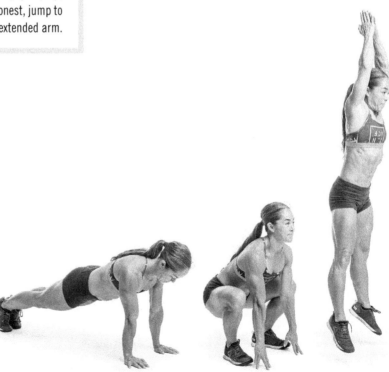

TRAINING WITH WEIGHTS

You could develop and execute a Firebreather program using exclusively body-weight movements. I've done this on numerous occasions when on military training deployments or when assigned to law-enforcement training academies where weights were not provided. Training with just body-weight movements is easy to fit into your life, and it's also cost effective. However, resistance training with weights and other tools can accelerate the development of power and also boost your efforts to add lean muscle mass and burn off body fat.

To access equipment, you'll need a gym of some kind. You can join a gym or can build your own garage gym (see page 84). You can begin with just a medicine ball and kettlebell, but you'll eventually need access to barbells, racks, dumbbells, and a pull-up bar. Rowing machines are great, and you'll want a rope to climb. CrossFit gyms will have all of this; conventional gyms may or may not be as well equipped.

Let's start with the basic skills necessary to use free weights smartly and safely.

BREATHING AND LIFTING WEIGHT

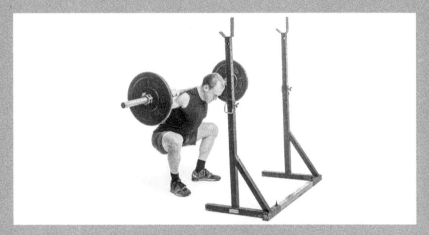

Breath awareness in weight lifting is imperative. Rolf Gates, renowned yoga teacher, once told me in relation to a yoga pose, "The breath moves the body." I really like this concept and utilize this philosophy in gymnastics, weight lifting, and yoga, with profound results. The key with the breath is to create pressure in the body, which produces force and tension. To create pressure, breathe in, filling yourself with life force. As your body begins to exert force into the weight, slightly breathe out, as if you were hissing. Make the sound a boxer might make upon absorbing an opponent's blow: a short, sharp exhale, which increases inner abdominal pressure.

Let's use the back squat as an example. At the top of this lift, I take in a deep breath to expand my lungs and pressurize my body. Keeping the breath in, I lower through the squat to the bottom position. As I start to apply force to the bar and extend my legs, I time my exhalation to match my ascent. The moment that I experience any resistance in my ascent, I focus on my breath and press the air out, which increases the pressure and force I can apply. At the top of the lift, I take a deep breath in and repeat the process.

It's important to breathe in when the body is upright and in the most advantageous position. In the deadlift, I take a deep breath in when I am standing. Holding that breath, I lower to the bottom position and address the bar. I might take one more sip of air to increase pressure, then begin my lift. As I stand up with the weight, I press the air out, increasing the force of my exhalation to match the resistance of the lift.

RACK MOVEMENT

The back squat and front squat begin with an often overlooked and important skill: removing the barbell from the rack, walking backward with it, and preparing to squat. When I train with new athletes, we isolate and practice this skill over and over until it's second nature. I stress that the lift begins the moment your hands address the bar. Part of developing mindfulness and adding a spiritual quality to your training program is learning to bring awareness to every step of a skill. Although taught here from the perspective of the back squat, the same principles apply with the front squat, or using the rack to perform a pressing movement.

1 Establish a grip on the barbell that is approximately three inches outside shoulders. The goal is to find a width that allows you to externally rotate your shoulders to create tension in your upper back, traps, and shoulders. You want to create a muscle shelf to rest the barbell on. Keep your wrists straight, elbows under shoulder. Thumbs can be either hooked over or under bar, whichever lends itself to wrist alignment.

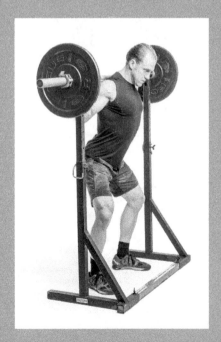

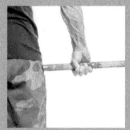

HOOK GRIP

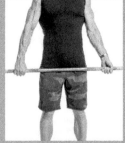

REVERSE GRIP

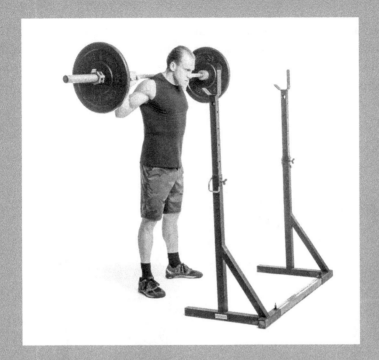

2 With muscle shelf set, step underneath barbell and engage the
bar. Pull the bar down onto your shelf, and simultaneously press
deltoids, traps, and upper back into bar. Create inner abdominal
tension by taking a deep breath in, and then squat barbell out of rack,
using legs, hips, and back at the same time. Keep neck neutral and
back straight.

3 With the weight on your back, take one step to the rear to clear the
rack. This step should be slow, accurate, and deliberate. Note: Step
the same way in and out of the rack every time to build muscle memory.
I always move my right foot first, then left. Take only one step back to
clear the rack, and trust yourself. There is no reason to look down at foot
placement. Develop the ability to feel yourself in space and time.

4 After completing your set of squats, return to the rack in the
same fashion. Deliberately step the right foot forward, then the left.
Set up over rack pins, and then squat the barbell straight down onto
the pins.

BACK SQUAT

>> After moving the bar out of the rack and establishing your stance, it's time to squat. The back squat is performed in much the same manner as the air squat. I teach and advocate the high-bar back squat, because it is easy to learn and transfers to the mechanics of the air squat. The barbell back squat is in the **open** category of movements.

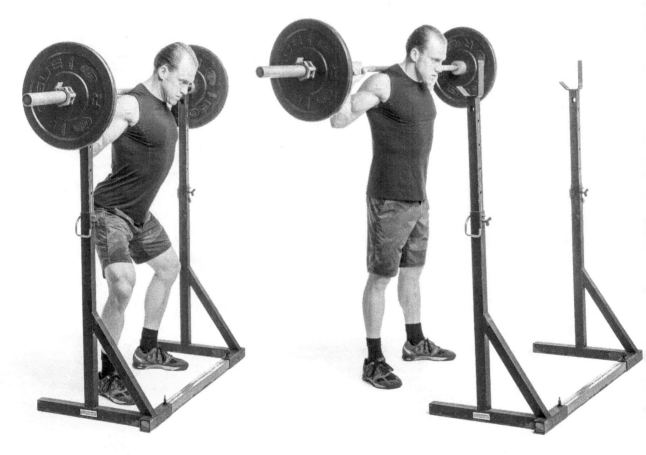

1 Squeeze butt, drive knees out, and imagine spreading the floor with your feet. You want a strong external rotation of feet and knees. Shoulders and upper back are tight, and you are maintaining your muscle shelf.

2 Keeping back flat and shins as vertical as possible, push butt back and down. Keep head and neck in alignment with spine.

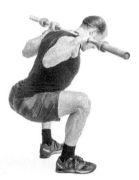

This angle highlights some of the essential elements of the back squat: Note that the crease of the hip is below the knees, scapula are externally rotated, wrists are straight, lumber curve is maintained, pelvis is in exterior rotation, knees are stacked over feet, neck is neutral, and barbell rests on the "muscle shelf" of upper traps and shoulders.

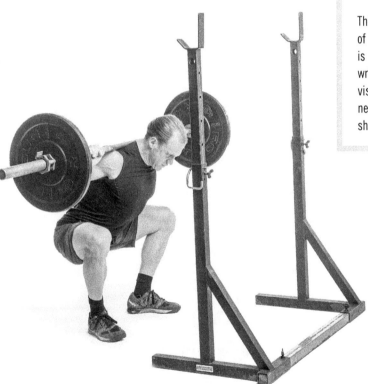

3 Keep tension in the entire body as you lower into the bottom position, bringing crease of hips below the knee. Remember the descent into any skill is not gravity fed; actively pull yourself into this position.

4 Driving through heels, extend legs and hip, returning to start position.

FRONT SQUAT

>> The back squat is a great conditioning tool. However, the front squat is an awesome "real world" type of skill. In the law-enforcement seminars that I teach, I correlate the front squat to lifting a suspect off the ground. We want to face our opponent, and generally speaking, when that same opponent is on our back, we have a problem. Lifting a child off the ground, picking up a bag of dog food, or hoisting a 5-gallon water jug—these are all examples of a front squat. The front squat belongs in the **open** category.

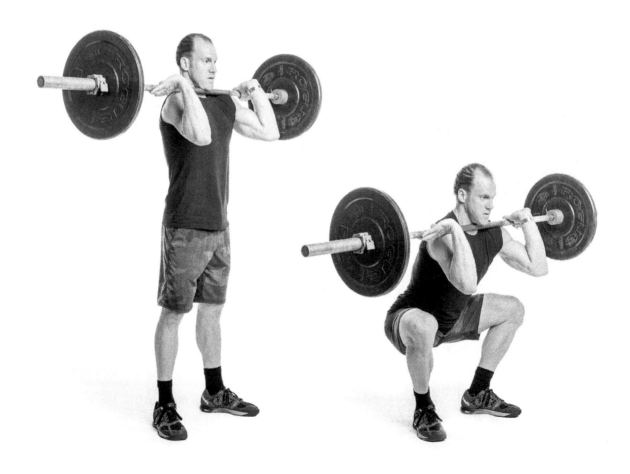

POINTS OF PERFORMANCE

The front squat is an "undercover" midsection development tool that can create exceptional strength through the core. Many times, following a front squat workout, the muscle soreness you experience is in the abdominal muscles. To really engage your core on this exercise, you'll need to create a strong sense of inner-abdominal pressure. This can be accomplished by taking a deep breath in through the nose just before the descent, holding the breath to the bottom position, then "pressing" the air out through a clenched jaw, making a hissing sound. Another great cue is to lead with the elbows as you return to the top position. This motion ensures a clean line of action and proper biomechanics.

1 Establish the front rack position. This can be accomplished using a rack, or through a power clean from the floor. The goal is to create a "muscle rack" or "muscle shelf" with your shoulders and upper chest supporting the bar, not relying on the strength of your arms. Wrap the thumb around the bar, as this transfers to ultimately lifting the load overhead. Imagine the elbows are laser beams, and you want to shine the laser directly in front of you.

2 Spread the floor with your feet, and create torque by a strong exterior rotation of the feet and knees. Squeeze your butt and engage through the midsection.

3 Keep your elbows pointed forward and up as you drive your knees out laterally, and push your butt back and down. Keep your chest as upright as possible. Keep the head and neck neutral and in alignment with your spine.

4 The bottom position brings the crease of your hip below your knee. Keeping the torso upright, lead with the elbows and drive out of the bottom position. Return to the top position through the same line of action as the descent.

OVERHEAD SQUAT

>> This is the king of the squatting movements, and like a microscope it will magnify any
fault in your air squat, back squat, or front squat. This skill takes years of practice, but the
athletic adaptation is well worth the time and effort. Start with a lightweight PVC pipe if necessary,
and spend at least 5 minutes each day practicing the range of motion. Add weight slowly and
gradually. The overhead squat is at the peak of the **open** category of skills.

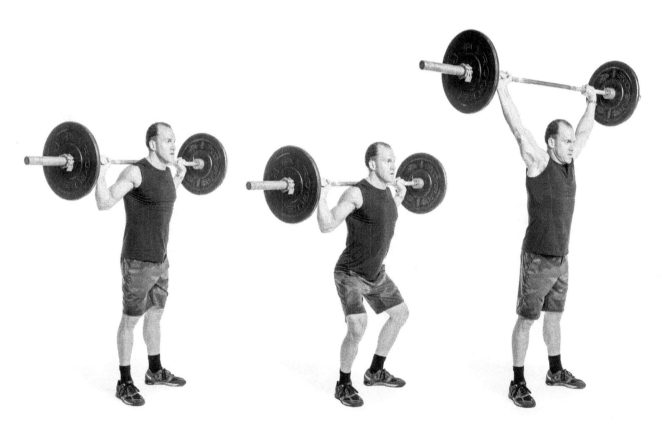

1 Using overhead squat grip-width (see Points
of Performance), engage barbell from rack.
Remove bar from rack and establish squat stance.

2 Driving knees out, pushing butt slightly
back, and keeping torso upright, load posterior
chain, referring to the back, butt, and
hamstrings.

3 Forcefully extend knees and hip, driving
barbell overhead. To maintain a stable shoulder
position, rotate armpits forward and imagine
you are trying to bend the bar in half. This creates
tension and torque. Rather than letting bar rest
on extended arms, actively press up into the bar.
Position bar in the center of palms, with wrists in
alignment with forearms. Do not bend wrists.

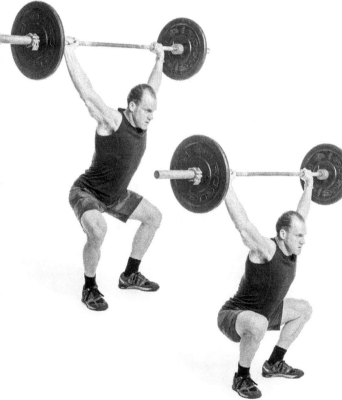

POINTS OF PERFORMANCE

Grip is key. To establish your grip, begin by using a PVC pipe and perform a series of pass-throughs: keeping arms extended, pass bar from hip to low back with grip as wide as possible. After each successful pass through, bring your hands a bit closer together and repeat. You are seeking a grip-width that allows for the pass-through to be successful, but where moving your hands even an inch closer together would require a bend in the arm. Then, use this grip on the PVC pipe, or transfer the grip to a barbell.

The overhead squat is a great test of midline stability and flexibility. For this reason, I use the overhead squat with new athletes as an assessment tool to test for motor control issues and mobility restrictions.

Note the bar evenly divides the body for the entire lift. In other words, the bar is always over the mid-foot. For this reason, it is important to pull the bar backward as the body descends. A common fault is to keep the bar "over the head" as opposed to slightly behind the head at the bottom of the squat.

5 The bottom position is the same as the air squat, back squat, and front squat. The crease of your hip is below knees, and chest is upright. Extend hips and knees and ascend to the top position.

4 Keeping shoulders engaged and pressing up into bar, push butt back and down, keeping torso upright. Focus on driving knees out and spreading the ground with your feet. As you descend, actively pull bar back to keep it over your center of mass.

6 If you are repeating multiple reps, reestablish top position. When concluding a set, guide weight to the ground in front of you. Do not attempt to receive anything heavier than an unloaded barbell on your cervical spine.

DEADLIFT

>> The deadlift is in the **open** category of skills. As Coach Glassman taught me, "It is unrivaled in its simplicity, yet unique in its capacity for increasing head-to-toe strength." The deadlift will improve any athletic skill. It is common both in the gym and in life: In the most advanced application, the deadlift is a prerequisite to the clean and jerk, and in its most basic application, the deadlift is nothing more than picking up an object off the ground.

Coach Glassman taught me the top-down setup technique, which I teach to this day. Empty-handed, you imagine lowering a loaded bar as you move into the start position onto the real bar. The moment your hands grip the actual bar, your back angle is already set (as in the photo), and you are correctly braced for the lift.

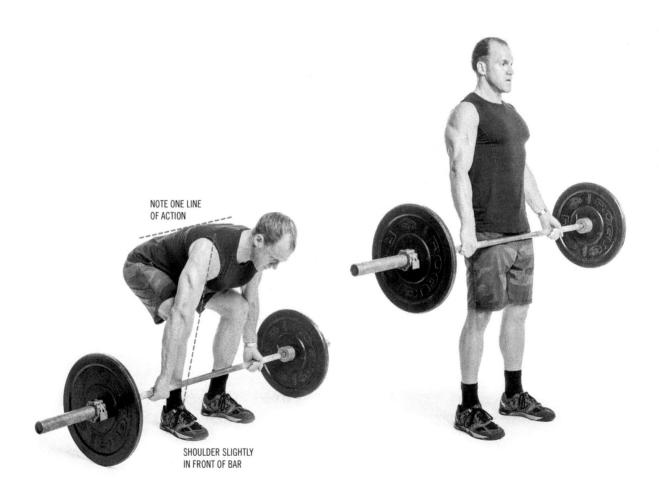

NOTE ONE LINE
OF ACTION

SHOULDER SLIGHTLY
IN FRONT OF BAR

POINTS OF PERFORMANCE

The key for the deadlift is the top-down set-up position. The moment your hands grip the bar, the body should be set and in position to engage the bar, and begin the lift. Trying to adjust the body with any significant movement when in the bottom position can be challenging in the least, and often times, prevent the athlete from the proper mechanical position needed to move a heavy barbell.

1 Lower to bar through a deadlift sequence, referring to the top-down principle. Grip bar and create as much tension in the body as possible.

2 Grip bar utilizing a reverse grip (see Grips, page 42). This grip is powerful and ensures minimal rotation of the bar in your hand. You can also employ a traditional weight lifting grip, which is the grip used for your clean. This grip is excellent for developing hand strength and pulling power for the clean.

3 Feet are straight and hip-width apart. Shins are vertical and knees are behind barbell. Head is down, allowing for one line of action from top of hip to crown of head.

4 Lift weight straight off the ground, keeping shoulders actively engaged and keeping barbell as close to the body as possible. At the start of the pull, the position of your spine remains unchanged.

5 Keeping barbell actively engaged and close to the body, stand up with bar, engaging glutes. Shoulders and hips rise at the same rate.

6 To lower barbell, return along the same line of action. Keep tension in the body the entire time, with legs extended until bar crosses knee. Or simply drop the bar from the top.

KETTLEBELL SWING

>> The kettlebell swing is in the **open** category. This is important to note, as a common fault
is to push the kettlebell with the arms. Power from the skill comes from the hips, not the
arms. My first CrossFit workout involved the kettlebell swing, and I was immediately hooked.
I incorporate the kettlebell in my own training, and I program this skill on a regular basis at my
gym. Note that most of the skills you can perform with a barbell or dumbbell can be performed
with a kettlebell.

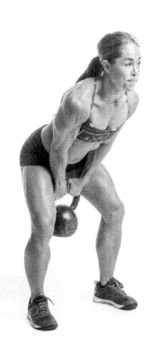

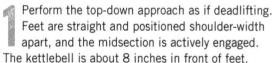

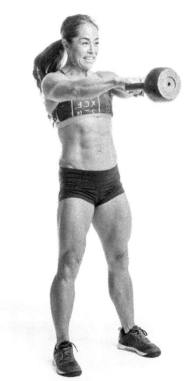

1 Perform the top-down approach as if deadlifting.
Feet are straight and positioned shoulder-width
apart, and the midsection is actively engaged.
The kettlebell is about 8 inches in front of feet.

2 Keeping shoulders pulled back, shins vertical,
and head neutral, press butt back and down to
engage hamstrings. Keep back flat and head
down to allow for a single line of action from top of
hip to crown of head.

3 At the bottom of the deadlift, reach hands
forward to grip kettlebell. Create as much
tension though body as possible.

4 Stand up through a deadlift sequence while
pulling or hiking the kettlebell, like a football,
back and between legs to begin the swing.

5 Actively extend leg and hip through triple
extension and drive hip forward. Keep arms
extended through this phase of the swing.

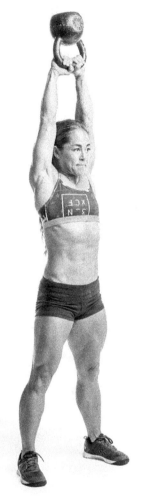

POINTS OF PERFORMANCE

The hike principle of initiating the first swing is a key nuance of the skill. The key with the swing is to understand the perfect bottom position. Keeping torso as upright as possible, slightly bend knees and bring extended arms to knees. Then, keeping arms extended, bring wrists between legs as if in the bottom position of the swing. Do not change back position or leg position. This is the ideal bottom position of the swing. The key is to engage the posterior chain and hip, and not the quads.

SCALING

Start with a light weight and take the necessary time to learn the proper mechanics and technique. Another scaling option is to swing the kettlebell only to eye level, known as the "Russian Swing." This would be appropriate for an athlete with limited shoulder mobility. Over time, gradually increase the height of the swing, until the full overhead range of motion is achieved.

6 As kettlebell approaches eye-level height, bend arm slightly. Think of the arm position as driving position; it's not fully extended, but not short like Tyrannosaurus rex arms either.

7 Using the power of the hip extension, continue to swing kettlebell overhead. Engage grip to point kettlebell straight up.

8 To cycle into the next swing, keep torso upright as you bring kettlebell down along the same line of action. As the kettlebell approaches hip level, actively push hips back, squeeze butt, and pull kettlebell back between legs. The descent of the kettlebell is active, not a gravity-fed movement. You are actually trying to beat gravity at advanced stages of application.

PRESS

>> The press is a classic **push** category skill, and a foundational strength movement if there ever was one. It's not just a shoulder exercise. Notice in the instructions that you are asked to squeeze the glutes. This action fires up all of the muscles of your trunk and core. Properly done, the press draws on muscles and motor patterns throughout the upper body and trunk.

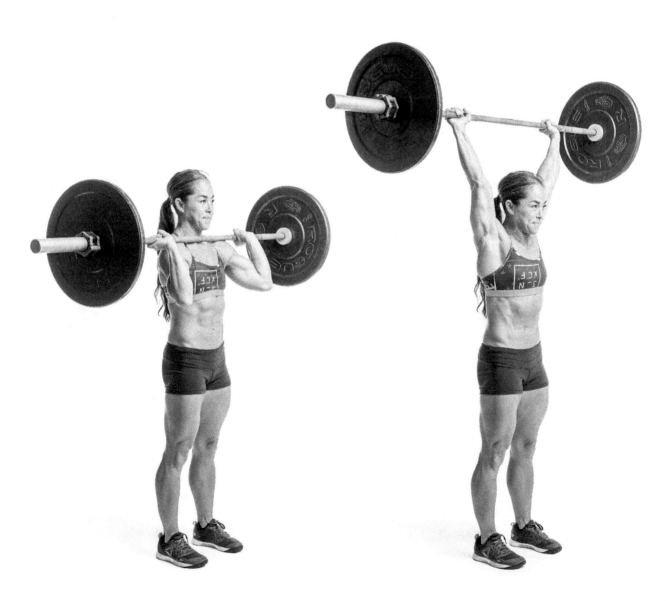

POINTS OF PERFORMANCE

Be sure to actively engage and brace through the midline. Keeping inner abdominal pressure during the press allows you to transfer energy from the mid-section through the shoulders and arms, and into the barbell. Maintaining midline stability becomes even more critical in the push press and push jerk, and must be fully developed on the press.

1 Engage bar in rack and establish your grip. Hands are just outside shoulders, with elbows slightly in front of bar. Bar rests in rack position, in the same manner as front squat. Thumb wraps around bar.

2 Step out of rack using the principles of the back squat or front squat. Feet are under hips, with toes pointing forward. Squeeze butt and engage midsection.

3 Press bar straight up while moving head slightly back to allow for a vertical bar path. As bar crosses face, continue to press bar straight up as head comes through. Repetition is complete when arms fully extend and bar is overhead.

4 Actively pull bar straight back down, following the same line of action as the ascent. Move head back to allow for a vertical bar path.

PUSH PRESS

>> The push press is in the **push** category of skills. It is a stepping stone, connecting the press to the Olympic lifting movements. In the push press, power travels from the hip and trunk muscles through the body's core-to-extremity chain, and that explosive energy pushes the bar overhead. Getting a good feel for this expression of power flow will transfer over into many other activities and sports.

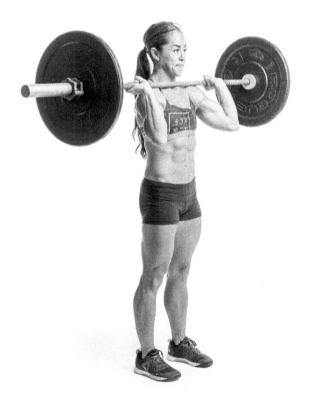

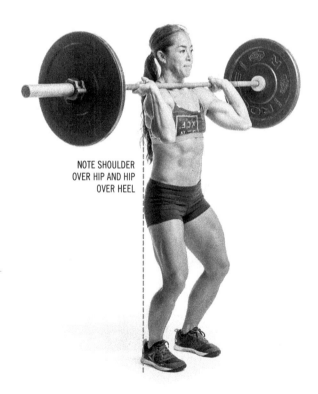

NOTE SHOULDER
OVER HIP AND HIP
OVER HEEL

1 Follow the same principles as the press for setup. In this lift, you will use hips and legs to create energy and momentum on the bar.

2 Keeping torso upright, drive knees out and press butt slightly back. Load hips as if you were preparing to jump straight up off the ground.

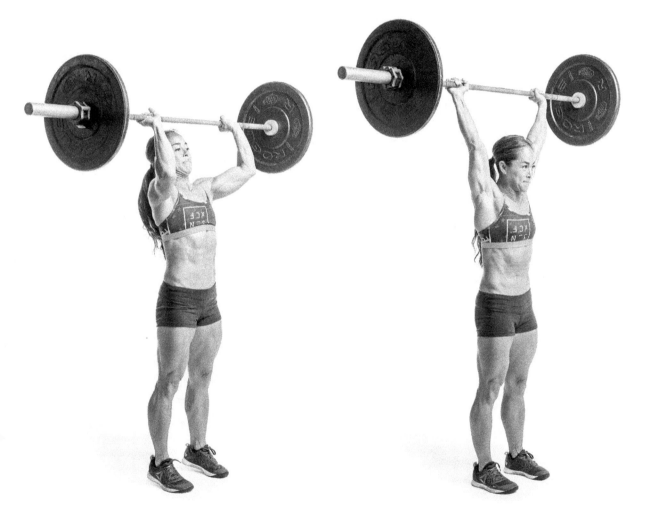

3 Forcefully extend legs and hips to transfer energy into barbell. Extend arms and capture the energy from the hip to follow through and press bar overhead. Move head slightly back to allow for a vertical bar path.

4 Due to the increased load this skill can move, as bar returns to rack position, use legs as shock absorbers to help receive the weight. After receiving the load, either reset the skill, or use the receiving position to immediately cycle another repetition.

BENCH PRESS

>> In athletic training, few things feel better than a well-executed set of bench press repetitions. Technique is key. Note: Always use a spotter. This is extremely important to your safety. The bench press is in the **push** category of skills.

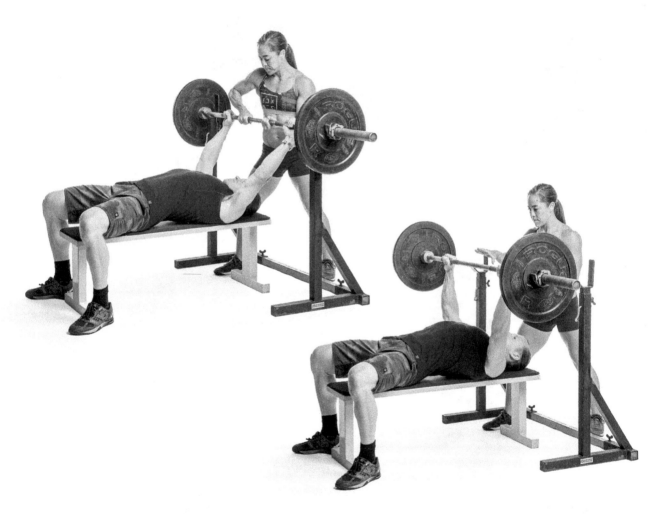

1 With the assistance of a spotter, bring bar off the rack. Set bar over sternum, remove "wobble" from the bar, then have spotter remove their hands. Take a deep breath in, and prepare for the lift.

2 With arms in extension, pull scapula back and down. Align barbell over sternum (not neck or chest). Feet are rooted into the ground, knees are driving out, shin angle is vertical. The points of contact with the bench are butt, shoulders, and head.

POINTS OF PERFORMANCE

The key is to engage the back when bench pressing, rather than focusing only on the chest. Imagine you are trying to bend the barbell in half as you press the bar. This action engages the latissimus muscles and helps to maximize engagement of the entire upper body. Body-weight push-ups are a good scale for the bench press.

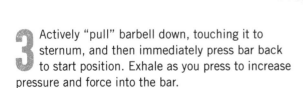

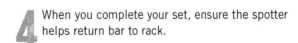

3 Actively "pull" barbell down, touching it to sternum, and then immediately press bar back to start position. Exhale as you press to increase pressure and force into the bar.

4 When you complete your set, ensure the spotter helps return bar to rack.

OLYMPIC LIFTS

>> The power clean, the clean, and the jerk are the three Olympic lifts in the Firebreather Fitness program. The power clean moves a barbell from the floor to the rack position (barbell resting across the front of shoulders). The clean is very similar to the power clean but involves a full front squat. The jerk is a complex motion that engages muscles throughout the body in a highly skilled explosive movement that drives the barbell upward while the athlete quickly drops and gets underneath. The clean and power clean are **open** category skills. With the addition of the jerk, the sequence encompasses both **open** and **push**. These are powerful exercises alone, but can also be combined into the clean and jerk (see sidebar, page 72).

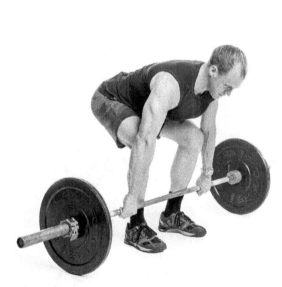
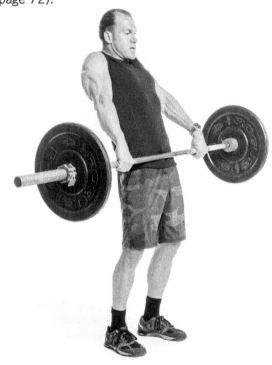

POWER CLEAN

1 Lower to bar through a deadlift sequence. Grip bar utilizing the hook grip, creating as much tension in the body as possible. In the hook grip, the pointer and middle finger "hook" over the thumb.

2 Feet are straight and hip-width apart, shins are vertical, and knee is behind barbell. Head is down to allow for one line of action from top of hip to the crown of the head.

3 Lift weight straight off the ground, keeping shoulders actively engaged, and keeping barbell as close to the body as possible. At the start of the pull, position of spine remains unchanged.

4 Keeping barbell actively engaged and close to body, continue to stand up with the bar, increasing bar's speed as it approaches the waist.

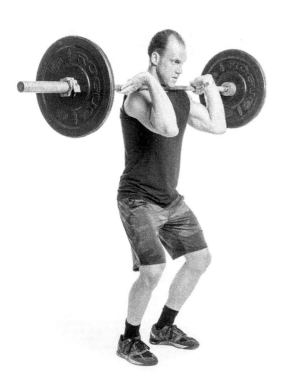

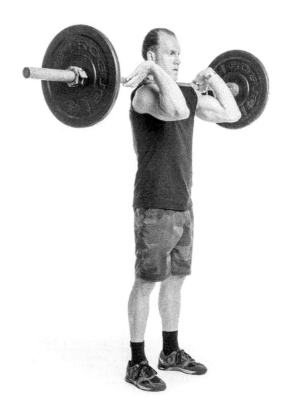

5 Once you have achieved triple extension (extension of ankle, knee, and hip), actively shrug shoulders.

6 In order to keep the bar's path vertical, pull elbows backward, and then quickly whip elbows forward, allowing barbell to come to rest on shoulders, known as the rack position. Note the slight re-bend of the knee and hip. The beauty of the power clean is the bar's continued acceleration

upward as the body retreats under the bar to catch it. Note elbows are facing forward and shoulders are over hips.

7 Stand all the way up with bar.

8 Return barbell along the same line of action to the floor.

JERK

1 Whether you take the bar out of the rack or are following a clean from the ground, the setup is the same. Engage through midsection, squeeze butt, and retract shoulders. Your elbows are positioned at 45 degrees, and your grip is either at or close to front rack position.

2 Keeping torso upright, push butt slightly back and down, drive knees out, and lower hips between feet. This phase of the dip is identical to the first four to six inches of your front squat and also identical to the dip position of the push press. Focus on keeping shoulders over hips.

3 Aggressively extend hips and knees into triple extension. This action will "jump" the barbell off your shoulders, similar to the action of the thruster (see page 74). As the bar clears your shoulders, pull head slightly back to allow for a vertical bar path.

4 As barbell travels upward, press yourself under bar. Catch barbell with arms fully extended, shoulders back, knees out and armpits forward.

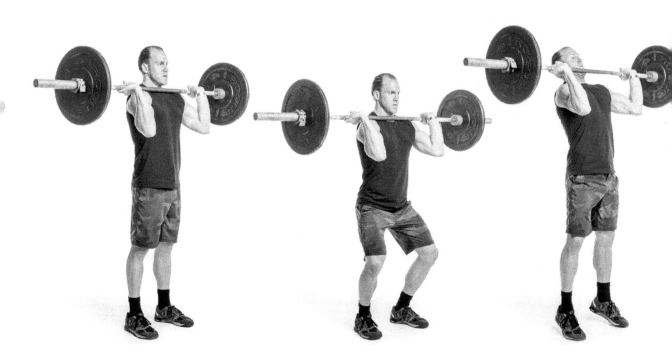

5 Overhead squat barbell to top position and reset feet if necessary. Repetition is complete with triple extension achieved through the ankle, knee, and hip, with arms fully extended and barbell overhead in frontal plane.

POINTS OF PERFORMANCE

With Olympic lifts, it's helpful to work with a good coach who can help you build the right patterns. Bad patterns and habits can be tough to shake. For drills and videos on the subject of Olympic lifts, go to www.firebreatherfitness.org.

Two bits of advice from Olympic lifting coaching great Mike Burgener are extremely helpful with the clean and jerk. One is "be a junkyard dog." This concept is all about aggressiveness. Sometimes you have to show that barbell who's boss, and get after it. The other is "when the arms bend, the power ends." Simply put, the arms are like hooks in this skill, and are just along for the ride. The power comes from the lower extremities and an aggressive shrug of the shoulders.

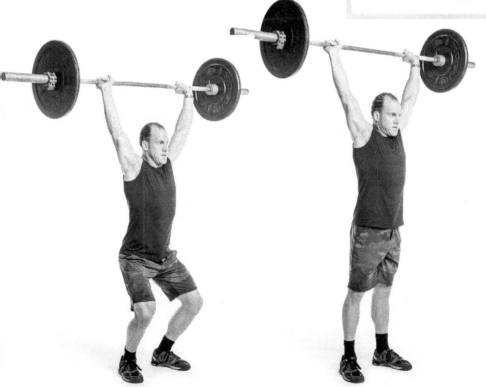

COMBINING THE
CLEAN AND THE JERK

The clean and jerk has the ability to greatly transform your athletic prowess and sense of strength. Approach the skill in two parts: First, nail a great clean, bringing the bar into your body's rack position. From that point you will probably need to reposition your feet under your hips and change your elbow position to achieve the setup position for the jerk. Then, following the steps on pages 70–71, take a deep breath and dip, drive, re-dip, and catch to complete the jerk.

The clean and jerk is a complicated exercise. When performed well, it's a thing of beauty. In a coordinated sequence of high-speed moves,

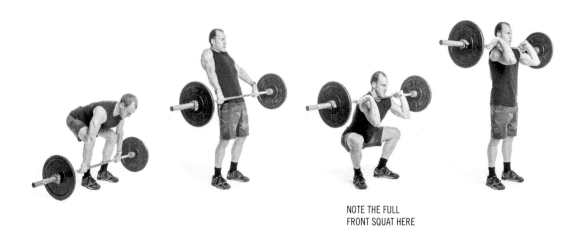

NOTE THE FULL
FRONT SQUAT HERE

you explosively lift the barbell from the ground and dive under it. With a challenging load, the clean and jerk demands equal parts physical prowess and courage. As weight lifting coach Mike Burgener says, "The best way to go after the clean and jerk is with the rabid mind-set of a junkyard dog." My point? Working hard at the clean and jerk pays dividends. Physical power is just the beginning; you'll also develop new reserves of determination, confidence, and mental toughness. A tip from Coach Burgener on how to achieve all of this: Bore through the fear by committing yourself absolutely to the task on hand, with a fanatical belief you'll get the job done. Use the clean and jerk as a skill to practice this attitude. Then spread it throughout your life.

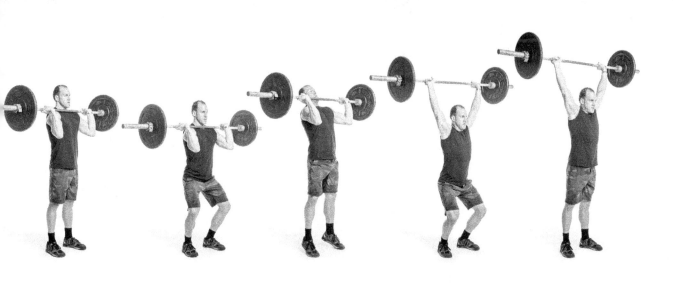

THRUSTER

The thruster combines an **open** and a **push** category into one seamless skill. However, the majority of the power in the skill will come through your open capacity. The thruster is a combination of a front squat and a push press. It engages so many muscles in a quick and repeatable action that this exercise packs a metabolic conditioning wallop like few others. In terms of the potential to maximize intensity, the thruster is hard to beat. At lighter loads, this skill can really accelerate the heart rate, and it develops great stamina and endurance. At heavier loads, the thruster develops amazing speed and explosiveness.

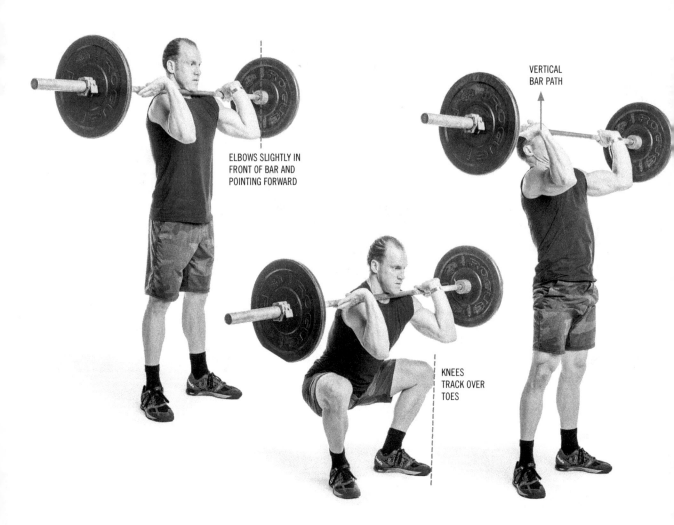

ELBOWS SLIGHTLY IN
FRONT OF BAR AND
POINTING FORWARD

VERTICAL
BAR PATH

KNEES
TRACK OVER
TOES

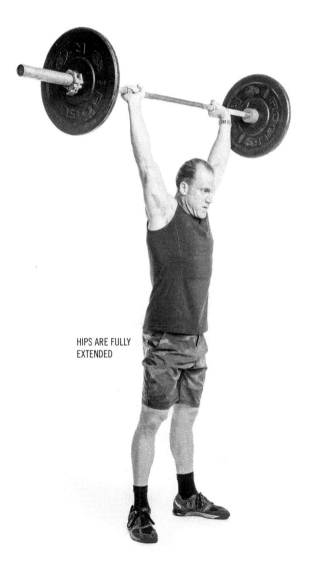

HIPS ARE FULLY
EXTENDED

POINTS OF PERFORMANCE

A great goal is 50 consecutive barbell thrusters with a 45-pound barbell for men, and a 35-pound load for women, in addition to a body-weight single-repetition thruster. One goal develops stamina and endurance; the other, strength and power.

A key detail is to ensure triple extension of the ankle, knee and hip, before the barbell leaves the shoulders. The principle here is to transfer energy through the rapid acceleration of the hip into the barbell, and this can only happen if the barbell is set in the rack position (on the shoulder) at the moment of extension.

1 Begin with barbell in rack position, with elbows slightly in front of bar.

2 Push butt back and down, keeping barbell in the frontal plane with elbows pointing forward. Chest remains upright, your weight is in your heels, and knees track over toes, as if you're spreading the floor with your feet.

3 Use full range of motion to bring the crease of the hips just below the knee. Pelvis remains in exterior rotation and thigh angle points up. Your weight remains in heels as knees track over toes.

4 Accelerate upward by contracting core, hips, and low back. Extend legs and hips, transferring energy into barbell. Once full extension of hip is reached, drive barbell overhead, fully extending arms. Notice bar remains in frontal plane.

5 Actively pull barbell back to rack position, keeping leg and hips fully extended until bar has reset on shoulders.

WALL BALL SHOT

>> The wall ball combines both an element of **open** and **push**, and develops accuracy, timing, coordination, and stamina. It combines the mechanics of the front squat and thruster, but adds an element of trajectory and follow through. This skill also teaches athletes how to receive an object that's propelled toward them, which has implications in martial arts and other athletic endeavors. Note: The traditional height of the wall ball target is 10 feet for men and 8 feet for women.

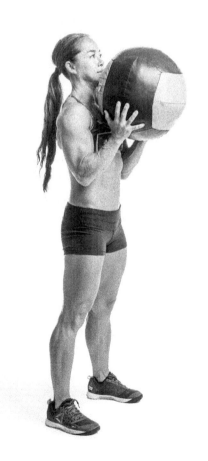

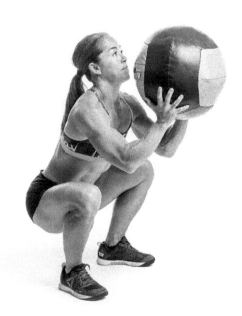

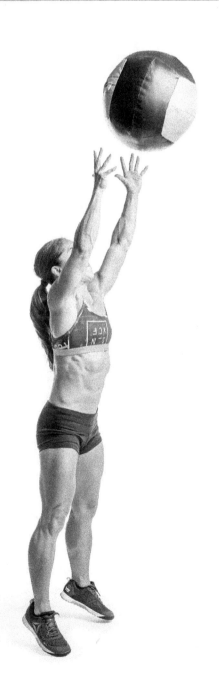

POINTS OF PERFORMANCE

Keep ball as high on torso as possible. This minimizes the distance ball has to travel to the intended target.

Receive ball as early as possible on the descent. By tracking ball early and controlling the final foot of its descent, you greatly increase the efficiency of the skill. Also, time the moment you press your butt back and down with the moment ball is in position on your chest. Guiding the ball into position helps cue the lower body in preparation for its descent.

1 In a squatting stance, engage medicine ball (10, 15, or 20 pounds) by pressing palms isometrically into ball. Keep wrists straight and elbows under wrists. Using the principles of the front squat, create a shelf with chest to support the load. Do not rely on arms to support the load.

2 Using the principles of the front squat or thruster, pass through a full range of motion squat. Elbows should remain vertical and angled between knees. Keep wrists straight.

3 Aggressively accelerate through the ascent of the squat. The moment you reach triple extension, transfer energy from the hip into the ball, and extend arms toward target. You are shooting the ball into the target.

4 Keep arms extended to receive ball. Pick up and track the ball as early as possible, guiding ball back to rack position. The moment the ball returns to a solid rack position, begin to push butt back and down to a squat, and then into the next repetition.

MASTERY

When it comes to a long-range and complete development of your fitness potential, it isn't just about repetition. It is about mastery.

If there's a secret to realizing your greatness as an athlete, it is investing in a long-term, deep practice of the basic skills in the program. Become obsessed with perfecting how you do a squat, a push-up, or a toes-to-bar movement. Imagine a great violinist who spends time each day practicing the fundamentals of playing his instrument. When he first learns the bow strokes, he doesn't check it off the list and move on to other things. He continues his practice. Golf is another solid example. Great golfers don't let a day go by without practicing their fundamental swings. When a top player's game begins to slide off the rails, she may start over at the very beginning, rebuilding her swing from the ground up.

The late Shotokan karate master Gichin Funakoshi was a great teacher of this lesson. Once he brought together one hundred of his finest students, black belts all, for a special training session. The martial artists crowded around waiting to hear the secret insight they were expecting from Funakoshi.

There was some confusion while they waited, because Master Funakoshi had dropped into what's called the horse stance, and with his right hand began silently executing an outward forearm block with his eyes looking straight ahead. Over and over, twenty repetitions, the karate master continued performing the movement.

Then his eyes moved and, as he continued performing outward forearm blocks, his eyes watched the workings of his arm, the rotation and the angles, transfixed. He continued in this manner for another 20 repetitions or more. Meanwhile, his students—all hoping for advanced instruction in karate—awaited the secret techniques that he would soon impart.

They were shocked when at last he spoke, saying: "I think I'm finally just starting to understand this technique."

In this short, cogent presentation, Funakoshi had delivered a remarkable lesson about what mastery truly is: a state of mind, riveted to a profound purpose, with an obsession to learn and free of the pull of ego.

My understanding of the path to mastery is grounded both in my martial arts training and in being coached by Greg Glassman. Coach frequently emphasized the concept of "virtuosity" in our approach to workouts. He used the word often, pressing us to execute movements with virtuosity. We all knew this had something to do with performing the movements skillfully, but one day after a workout I asked Glassman why this word had so much importance for him.

He related a story of a day years earlier when he had gone to watch a high school gymnastics competition in Los Angeles, in a large, packed gym. A number of gymnasts were performing routines throughout the competition venue, on parallel bars, a horse, on the rings, the balance beam, and the floor. It was noisy, but at one point a hush fell over the gym. He said it took him a moment to figure out what had caused the deep silence, and that he was expecting something very incredible.

The crowd had become mesmerized by a gymnast who was on the rings and holding a simple L-sit. He was gripping both rings with his hands, and holding himself up with his legs extended horizontally.

This fixation struck Coach as odd. After all, the L-sit is such a basic movement in gymnastics that you don't even get any points for doing it. The points come from executing more complicated movements. But Glassman figured out what the drama was all about: This gymnast was performing the L-sit incredibly well. The definition that Coach had for virtuosity was related to what he saw that day: doing the common thing uncommonly well.

Virtuosity \vər-chü-ʻä-sə-tē\ (n)
Doing the common thing uncommonly well

It was a simple position, one that gymnasts are introduced to on their first day of practice, but this athlete had an entire audience spellbound for reasons they may have had a hard time articulating. When a master performs a common act with uncommon skill, we seem to perceive it almost on a subconscious level.

I can't emphasize enough how valuable it will be for you in your training to come to each session with a burning desire to finish the session able to perform fundamental movements better—even if the improvement and understanding are infinitesimal. It's like laying one brick after another. You'll discover this attention to detail will reap great satisfaction and allow you to make progress you might not have thought possible.

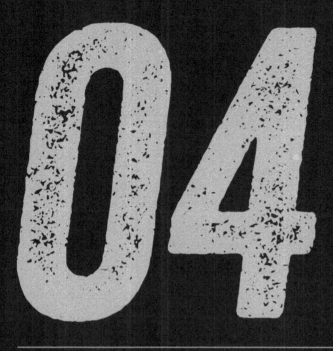

GETTING STARTED

THERE WERE SIX OF US sprawled across the floor after performing a timed workout using two movements with multiple sets and reps: a thruster (a blend of front squats and push presses) and a pull-up. On the whiteboard that morning, it didn't stand out in any way. But this thruster–pull-up workout (later named "Fran"—to simply communicate benchmark workouts, Coach Glassman assigned them names) had pushed us into the redline territory of extreme physical exertion and banging into and over the anaerobic threshold. It was a scorcher of a workout, literally and figuratively, as each of us looked at one another and noticed how our throats had been seared by the breathing and metabolic intensity that comes with an all-out effort.

"It felt like I was breathing fire the entire time!" I proclaimed in a raspy voice. "It's like we're a bunch of firebreathers!"

That word stuck, and in the years since "Firebreather" has come to describe more than just the effects of a hard workout. Being a Firebreather means that you bring all of your energy, spirit, and intent to your training—you burn with purpose and give it your absolute best.

We defined Firebreather in Chapter 2. But let's look at it a little bit closer—there are two parts to being a Firebreather.

1. One who faces the triumphs and tribulations of great physical opposition with an indomitable spirit.

To be a Firebreather, you take on this opposition by training as if your life depends on it. When you make that kind of commitment, incredible amounts of energy and ability will be realized. I faced opposition in my jobs in law enforcement and military service. But opposition can also refer to the trials and tribulations that come with taking on any significant goal.

2. An optimistic energy associated with the heart of an athlete.

The "heart of an athlete" is key. Think about approaching your workouts and your life as a professional athlete. Even if you have only an hour (or less) to invest in your physical, mental, and spiritual training each day, approach it with the energy and focus of an Olympic athlete. Pour your heart into your training, focus on the effort you put into each workout, and the results will astonish you.

Training in order to realize your full physical and athletic potential begins with having a rock-solid athletic foundation. As a first responder, I needed a physical fitness training program that would prepare me for anything and everything on any given moment of any given day. A sound athletic foundation does that.

An athletic foundation is also the target if your mission is to train for life. Peter Attia, MD, an expert in longevity and nutrition, makes the case that life is what we should be training for in the first place. To make life your sport—to be the best parent you can be, to do the best job you can in your work, to sustain full mobility and independence into your 70s, 80s, and 90s—is the real goal.

If sheer athletic performance in a specific sport, such as running a marathon or playing in a soccer league, is what's most important to you, then an athletic foundation is also key. While it is true that if you want to reach your potential in a specific sport, then sport-specific training is essential, it is also true that you'll be able to go higher and farther by first developing your athletic foundation.

A strong foundation goes well beyond the physical, of course. The complete expression of your potential as an athlete, a student, a professional, a first responder, a spouse, a parent, or whatever combination best represents you, demands that you strive to train not just body but also mind and spirit. In this chapter we'll focus on the physical, weaving in the layers of mental and spiritual training in later sections of the book.

THE 21-DAY FIREBREATHER FITNESS PROGRAM

I created the Firebreather Fitness program with the intention of making your workouts simple, sustainable, effective, efficient, and fun!

Limited time in the day is a given for most of us. In military and law-enforcement work, there is no such thing as an 8-hour workday, and the same can be said for so many professions—doctors, teachers, executives, parents. There are already myriad responsibilities demanding your time and energy. You want and need a high-performance training plan that can be easily incorporated into your everyday routine.

Because this program is made of up high-intensity workouts, most of your workouts will range between 8 and 20 minutes in duration, and only rarely will they take longer than 30 minutes. Believe me when I say that 8 minutes of high-intensity exercise is far more effective than an hour of bopping around a gym doing a few sets of bench presses here and there.

When you work out this way, it frees up *more* energy and productivity for your daily life. You will see the difference for yourself in a matter of weeks.

The Firebreather Fitness program makes use of basic gym equipment. For years, the fitness world gravitated toward expensive weight machines, like Nautilus and Cybex. These machines were designed to isolate individual muscles. The technology to deliver this concept grew ever more expensive and complicated in motorized resistance machines with embedded computers.

I've seen and tried a variety of fitness programs, and I can say with confidence: Basic equipment produces better results. A pull-up bar or set of gymnastics rings is far more effective than an expensive cable-crossover machine. Yes, you read that correctly: The bar at the local playground is more valuable to you as a Firebreather than the machines crowded into a conventional gym. There are a number of basic gymnastics movements requiring nothing more than body weight for resistance that will get you into phenomenal physical condition. Don't underestimate the power of these exercises.

This program also incorporates weights in classic lifts like bench press, squats, and thrusters. It's the combination of functional movements, both the body-weight exercises and those where you are working against heavy resistance, done at high intensity—that will make you a Firebreather.

EQUIPMENT

To do the Firebreather Fitness program, you need good, basic training equipment. If feasible, build a home gym. Consider buying used equipment in order to keep spending low. A scuffed-up 45-pound plate works just as well as a shiny new one, at a fraction of the cost. Craigslist can be a useful source for building a great home gym. Here is what you need:

Barbell: Men should use a 45-pound bar, and women a 35-pound one, with appropriate sizing of the grip width.

Weights: Assorted weights are available for your barbell. You can start with just a few and then add to your collection as your strength and power develops. Dumbbells can be used in place of weights or a kettlebell if your budget is strict.

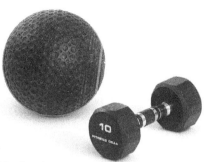

Medicine ball: Ten-pound medicine balls are good for beginners. From there you can work up to 15-pound or 20-pound medicine balls.

Box: Women should start with a 16-inch box and progress to a 20-inch, and men should start with a 20-inch box and progress to a 24-inch.

Gymnastics rings: One of the most versatile pieces of equipment around. You can throw them over a tree branch and do pull-ups, ring dips, and ring rows, and they'll let you begin working on advanced moves like the muscle-up.

Pull-up bar: Gyms typically have an apparatus for pull-ups. If you want to invest in a garage gym, you can find ceiling or wall mounts online. Or you can put a pull-up bar across your doorframe. Alternatively, you can get creative and find bars for pull-ups at playgrounds or outdoor fitness trails.

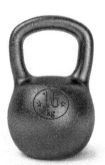

Kettlebell: A good starter weight for men is 35 pounds; women should start at 25 pounds. Ideally, you'd have a range from 25 to 53 pounds.

Jump rope: This can be as simple as a length of rope from the hardware store, or you can choose from a variety of jump ropes at the sporting goods store.

Squat rack: A squat rack is great to own. The higher priced ones even come with a built-in pull-up bar. Or you can buy basic squat stands for less than $100. But a higher quality rack is worth the investment. I recommend checking Craigslist if you don't want to buy new. Scratches have no negative impact on its usefulness.

Rower: The Concept2 rower has become the fitness industry standard. It is lightweight, easy to store, and a potent piece of exercise equipment. You can buy one new for less than $1,000.

If a home gym isn't possible for you, then get creative! You could, for example, keep a mobile gym in your car. Pack rings, dumbbells, kettlebells, jump rope, and a medicine ball, and find a park to work out in. I know several athletes who take this approach, driving to a variety of outdoor locations throughout the week to work out. At my gym in Santa Cruz, I have a 12-passenger van that I load up with gear, and take members to the beach or hills to work out. When you develop the "eye of a Firebreather" the world becomes your gym!

If you have access to a gym with free weights and a pull-up bar, you can do the program. You may need to innovate at times to do the workouts. If, for example, a workout calls for running, thrusters, and pull-ups, then you might have to figure out a plan where you can use a barbell or dumbbells for the thrusters near a pull-up bar so that you prevent others from taking over a piece of equipment in the middle of your session. If it's impossible to run outside or jump on a treadmill for the runs, then you can substitute in a similar activity, like rowing, or something as simple as air squats.

Most fitness programs fall short because they don't offer the level of precision and personalization that you would get from a coach. Rather than having, for example, a shirt tailored just for you, it's more like one size fits most: the results will be mixed. My mission is to give you a set of tools to drive you rapidly toward a state of highly tuned physical fitness. These tools allow you to customize the 21-day program to your current state of fitness.

TOP 10 LESSONS
FOR BUILDING A GARAGE GYM

1 **Conceal or store off-site any non-essentials to the gym.** These are things like your water heater, Christmas boxes, etc.

2 **Invest in rubber floor covering.** Doing so is vital to creating the finished and professional look of a gym and prolongs the life of your equipment.

3 **Add some motivation to the walls.** Hang affiliate shirts, photographs, posters—anything that provides inspiration for you.

4 **Build a library.** Select books that offer education and inspiration, and refer to them often.

5 **Install a whiteboard.** It should be part of every gym and provides a surface on which to capture workout times, chart progress, diagram workouts, and write fun quotes.

6 **Lead by example.** Work out in public places. Run down your street. Invite your neighbors over for coffee and teach them how to squat!

7 **Be clean and tidy.** Because of the limited space of a residential gym, everything must have a place. Keep the gym pristine—it is a reflection of you and your attention to detail.

8 **Refer to the "garage" as a "gym."** Words are important. You should associate your workout space with a true gym, not just a garage.

9 **Choose quality over quantity.** Make the investment in safe, durable equipment you can be proud of.

10 **Create a sense of gym ownership for yourself and the friends you train with.** Make others feel at home in your gym.

Adapted from Greg Amundson, "Garage Gym 101," *CrossFitJournal* (2010), journal.crossfit.com.

PRACTICING VIRTUOSITY

To be successful, every workout must be focused on achieving these three things:

1 **Good technique.** Learning how to do the movements properly is not an overnight process. Practice and perfect them. Technique also includes range of motion, which naturally lends itself to the next point, intensity.

2 **High intensity.** With good technique intact, maintaining a high level of intensity and effort will pay off, delivering metabolic stimulus and adaptation. Every workout is set up with time as a critical component. You are either doing as much work as you can in a given time, or completing a piece of work in the least amount of time possible. The element of time is critical to the Firebreather program.

3 **Consistency.** Schedule workouts in such a way that there is no danger of them being trumped by other things. Early mornings are a good time for many people, before others are awake and start making demands on their time. Get it done! It's a great way to start the day. If early mornings aren't an option for you, then commit to working out at a specific time of day.

Consistent, high-intensity efforts using functional movements and good form are the secret to long-term, steady progress.

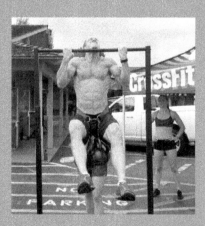

A weighted pull-up demonstration outside of CrossFit Amundson in Santa Cruz, California— proper technique is key!

THE MASH-UP TEST

Both a workout and also a time trial, the mash-up test is a way to get real-time information on where your fitness stands so that you can chart your overall progress as well as dial in the optimal workout load and intensity for the day.

THRESHOLD TRAINING

Many people preparing to do a workout have a problem: figuring out how much to do and how hard to go. Firebreather threshold training is designed to take the guesswork out of determining that load. A short test before key workouts will let you know exactly what your training intensity (reps or weight) should be for each movement.

Mash-up tests will help you find out how many reps you can do of a specific movement in one minute. Each test includes two or three movements.

To explain, let's take a look at a basic mash-up test: jump-rope double unders and kettlebell swings. You will do a one-minute test of each movement to get an accurate data point on your fitness and skills.

First, count the number of double unders you can do in one minute. Start the clock and do as many as you can before that minute is up. Beginner athletes can do traditional single jumps.

Record the total number of repetitions completed in a journal or on the whiteboard. Rest 1 minute to recover.

Next, see how many kettlebell swings you can do in 1 minute. Record the number of reps completed.

Take 1 minute to recover.

What's next?

Following your 1-minute recovery, take 2 minutes and determine the threshold percentage to use in the workout. During the initial stages of the 21-day Firebreather Fitness program you will be training at 30 to 40 percent of your maximum capacity achieved on the 1-minute test.

For example, let's say you did 100 double unders and 30 kettlebell swings in the mash-up. Multiply these numbers by 40 percent, or 0.4, each. You get:

40 double unders
12 kettlebell swings

Plug these numbers into the 7-round workout of the day, which totals 14 minutes. At the start of minute one, you do 40 double unders. Rest the remainder of the minute until minute 2 begins, then start your first set of 12 kettlebell swings. After the 12 swings, put down the kettlebell, pick up the rope, and wait until minute 3 begins to start the next set of double under repetitions.

Every odd minute you're on the jump rope, and every even minute you're swinging the kettlebell. The 14-minute workout is written like this:

Every Minute on the Minute (EMOM) for 14:00 (7 rounds of each):
Odd min. = 40% threshold for jump rope
Even min. = 40% threshold for kettlebell swing

1-REP MAX TESTS

For the strength-specific components in the plans, you will need to find your 1-rep max for different movements. So when the program instructs you to "find your 1-rep max deadlift," you will work toward the most you can lift with the given movement in a safe, controlled, and skilled manner. Knowing what a 1-rep max is for a certain weight movement will allow you to work on that movement with more reps, using specific percentages of your max.

Consider the thruster. On day 3 of the 21-day advanced plan, you'll start your workout by figuring out what your 1-rep max is with thrusters. At the end of the test, you will see this set:

---

5 thrusters (60% 1RM)

If your 1-rep max on the thruster was 100 pounds, day 3 of the advanced plan would require you to perform 5 thrusters with 60 pounds during the workout.

PROGRESSION

Within each week, the program will offer workouts where the percentage increases to bring the athlete closer to the threshold. This promotes adaptation. The mash-up and 1-rep max tests make the program more flexible. As strength and fitness grows, the reps/weight will increase.

As mentioned, the plans also include standard baseline workouts, strength-specific components, and Fitness Outside the Box activities.

The schedules in the back of the book can certainly be followed as is, but they can also serve as templates for you to use in building your own individual program. After you progress through the program, work in some new movements. Be creative and intuitive. Or step it up to the next level—beginner to intermediate to advanced. Most of all, make it an adventure. The more spirit and fun you infuse into your training, the more you'll get out of it (and the more likely you are to stick with it).

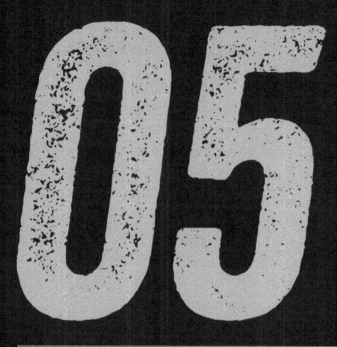

TAKE IT OUTSIDE

ONE RUT I WANT YOU TO AVOID is doing all of your training inside a gym. I feel so strongly about this that I have designed the Firebreather Fitness programs with it in mind. Built into the 21-day training plans are assigned workouts that say: "Fitness Outside the Box."

Getting outside has innumerable health benefits. Perhaps the most vital health benefit from being outside is adequate sun exposure. Many Americans suffer from a deficiency in vitamin D—also known as "the sunshine vitamin." Some three-quarters of Americans are reported to be deficient in this nutrient. Scientists are beginning to connect the dots between the risk of heart disease and cancer when it comes to a lack of the sunshine vitamin, as well as linking low vitamin D intake to bone-density loss and rickets.

Less tangible health connections to taking your workouts to the back yard, a beach, or a local park include the dimensions of spiritual and mental health. Being outside is just plain fun. Doing all of your training inside a gym can be a drag on you. Fresh air, sunshine, new places to be and train—all of this is psychologically restorative and spiritually powerful. Get on a bike, hike up a trail, go for a swim, find a field and throw down with body-weight exercises, put on inline skates, surf, ski, paddleboard, or even just go for a walk downtown.

Some of the activities I lead and advocate at my own gym are hill running, stair sprints, and running on a variety of terrains, such as sand, dirt, grass, and trails. Many general physical skills, such as accuracy, coordination, agility, and balance, are best developed during outdoor activity, on a less forgiving surface than an even and consistent rubber gym floor. Running a trail involves hundreds of microcorrections of the knee, ankle, and foot, and requires a heightened sense of sight and an awareness of your surroundings. And while this quality of precision of movement can certainly be applied in the gym, it cannot be learned in the gym.

Some of my favorite exercises and workouts can easily be performed outdoors. For example, an assortment of push/pull and open/close movements can be done at a playground, using bars, steps, and benches. All of this is good stuff, activating different motor patterns in your body and muscles you might not even have known you have.

Fresh air, sunshine, new places to be and train—all of this is psychologically restorative and spiritually powerful.

Changing things up in your routine is a potent recipe for promoting performance gains. It's not just a matter of changing the workout; it's exploring and experiencing all the variables. Different levels of heat, elevation, surface, and time of day are a few of the ways to add variety and keep body and mind in a state of development. And without a doubt, the spiritual impact of exercise in the sun, on the surface of the earth, is profound.

You are limited only by your imagination when it comes to getting outside of the box. Here are some of my favorites to get you started.

GREAT BODY-WEIGHT "FITNESS OUTSIDE THE BOX" WORKOUTS

The principles of the Firebreather Fitness program provide a framework for you to develop your own programming, adding your unique perspective, imagination, and intuition into your programming. Although the workouts below are some of my favorites, I encourage you to take what works and make changes where you feel they are necessary. I've also included some of my personal records on the workouts—in the event you're up for a challenge, try to best them!

STAIR CHASERS

Beginning at the bottom of the stairs, sprint to the first landing. At the first landing, turn around and sprint back to the bottom starting position. Without stopping, sprint up the stairs to the second landing, then turn around and sprint back to the start position. Continue until you reach the top of the staircase. One of my favorite locations for this workout is the wooden stairs at Seacliff State Beach in Aptos, California. From bottom to top, there are six landings. Note: This workout is best when your chosen staircase has multiple landings, but if all you have is a steep hill, you can do the same workout: Just use cones or markers to signify landings. This is a demanding workout. You may start with just one round, and then as you gain fitness, add additional rounds.

BURGENER GONE MAD
150 burpees for time

Named after the great Olympic lifting coach, Mike Burgener. This can be done anywhere—your local park would work just fine. You might start with a goal of performing 50 burpees in 10 minutes. Steadily work at it, and then up your goal to 80 or 100. Advanced Firebreathers will shoot for 150 in 10 minutes. Be sure to adhere to the points of performance on page 46 for the burpee.

SUPER SUN

3 rounds for time:
50 squats
Run 400 meters
30 push-ups

Following the first round, note your "split time" (the time it took you to complete one round). Try to keep your remaining two rounds within 30 seconds of that first round. Doing this workout at the beach is priceless. I've also varied this session by subbing an ocean swim for the run. I swim straight out into the ocean, and each time my right hand strokes through the water is "one rep." After I complete 40 reps, I turn around and swim back to shore. My best time on a soft-sand surface is 8:57.

ANYWHERE/ANYTIME

4 rounds for time:
Run 400 meters
50 squats

This was one of Coach Glassman's favorite outdoor workouts, and we conducted it on a variety of outdoor surfaces, from sand to grass. An extra challenge is to perform this workout on a hill, running up and down, and performing the squats at the bottom. My best time on this workout is 9:17.

SHUTTLE RUNS

EMOM, add a 10-meter sprint:
Min. one: sprint 10 meters
Min. two: sprint 20 meters, etc.

Sand presents a challenging surface for this workout. It's best on a 10-meter course, because ideally you are changing directions at the end of each sprint. I advocate touching one hand to the surface just beyond the cone or 10-meter line you've established. I performed this workout with UFC legend Gray Maynard at Pleasure Point Beach in Santa Cruz, California, on a regular basis. The goal is to work up to 7 rounds. Then, for a real challenge, when you can no longer maintain the interval, rest one full minute, then start over at your last successful interval, working back down to a 1×10-meter sprint.

TABATA SQUAT MASH-UP

A Tabata squat session consists of 20 seconds of squats followed by 10 seconds of rest, completed 8 times. Following the Tabata interval, rest for 10 seconds, then immediately perform as many reps of pull-ups (or push-ups, toes-to-bar, or whatever other exercise you choose) in 4 minutes. Your score is the lowest round of reps you are able to net in the Tabata sequence, multiplied by the total number of push-ups, pull-ups, etc. you completed. So if you were combining the Tabata squat with push-ups, and in the third round of your Tabata squat workout you got 10 squats, but you were able to get 11 in all of the others, you would multiply 10 (your lowest per round score) times the total number of push-ups completed, say 100. Therefore, your score would be 10×100 for a total of 1,000. Record this number in your journal. Choosing the lowest round of Tabata squats forces you to remain consistent during each round. Named after famed Japanese research scientist Dr. Izumi Tabata, Tabata workouts are extremely effective at building your endurance and stamina.

400-METER WALKING LUNGE

Measure a 400-meter distance using cones or other markers, then time yourself traveling that distance using only a walking lunge. (See the scaling options on page 27.) This workout is equal parts mental and physical. At first, it may seem like you are doing a lot of work, but not getting anywhere!

BLASTERS

Run 400 meters	Run 400 meters
100 push-ups	50 toes-to-bar
Run 400 meters	Run 400 meters
50 pull-ups	100 squats

This is one of my favorite workouts that covers all the principles of the open, close, push, and pull methodology. (Note: This workout requires a pull-up bar.)

~

THOSE ARE SOME IDEAS for vigorous training options; each can be scaled to your current level of fitness. If you want to make it even simpler, just put on running shoes and get out on the trails for an hour, hop on a mountain bike and explore, or learn a new sport you have always wanted to try. All of these will do wonders to energize and invigorate your training.

PLAY SPORTS

Have you ever wanted to learn to surf? Or do a marathon or an ultramarathon? Or join a soccer league? Do you think your exercise program gets in the way? Quite the opposite—the Firebreather Fitness plan is an optimal first step toward making your sports dream come true.

There are plenty of 12-week programs out there that promise to get you from the couch to the starting line of a marathon or triathlon. But here's the problem—without a general fitness foundation and a strengthened set of general skills, along with a knowledge of how to move well, you are going to struggle with the training. Also, when it comes to an activity with a lot of repetitive movements, not knowing how to move well can have adverse effects on your joints and body.

Firebreather Fitness plans address several general athletic skills: cardiovascular/respiratory endurance, stamina, strength, flexibility, power, speed, coordination, agility, balance, and accuracy. Together, these build in you a super-sound athletic foundation and will allow you to pick up a new sport more readily and enjoy it with less risk of acute or chronic injuries.

Furthermore, the converse is true: Taking on a new sport will do wonders for your fitness goals. It will energize your training with a new goal, and it will draw greater nuances from the general skills into your body and mind as what you learn will be fed back into your growing capacities.

I learned this the hard way.

In 2009, I hit a major snag during the qualification for the CrossFit Games. I had been training consistently for eight years and had continued to improve every year. I had put my training to use in various roles, including serving in the Army and as a SWAT operator with the sheriff's office in Santa Cruz. I considered myself well prepared for the unknown and the

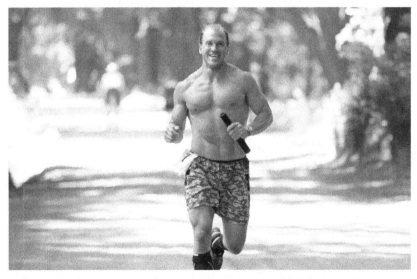

During a 5K race in the forest of Aptos, California. Outdoor running has a spiritual quality to it that I love.

unknowable. I had even been dubbed the "Original Firebreather." Given all this, qualifying for the Games was surely in my wheelhouse.

But there's always a reality check in the pursuit of preparing for the unknown and unknowable. It's always ready to put you to the test and weed out weaknesses in your training program. It will keep you humble.

As it did with me in 2009.

Despite having plenty of strength, power, stamina, and an assortment of skills in the gym, I had my Achilles' heel: double unders. I didn't like doing them and, because I let that get in the way of my judgment, I hadn't practiced them and mastered them. This was a costly mistake, and it bit me in 2009 when a workout to qualify for the games was comprised of deadlifts (no problem!) and double unders, a jump-rope movement where the rope passes beneath your feet two times per swing. The double-under nature of this movement ramps up the cardiovascular demand and taxes a range of skills.

I'll jump to the painful conclusion here: Despite an all-out effort, I couldn't do the double unders well enough to qualify. I fell short. As one of the early leaders of the CrossFit movement, this was embarrassing.

I could draw a line from my inability to perform this movement directly to an ego conflict. Ego often leads us to choose workouts that we like and are good at, and urges us to avoid movements that we don't feel confident with.

My failure at what had become a routine skill in CrossFit offered me a potent and valuable lesson.

When I did not qualify for the Games that year, I went back to the drawing board and worked hard to improve my double unders. In a matter of weeks I had become adept at them. All it took was intention and consistent attention, and an obsession to learn a skill.

But here the story took an unexpected and powerful turn. Because I had addressed a deficiency in my set of basic skills—in this case, my coordination and accuracy, honed by the double unders—the adaptations the training incurred spread throughout my athletic capacity. Indeed, my entire athletic foundation took a leap forward, and skills outside of the purely athletic realm also got a bounce.

For example, I noted that my skills on the shooting range jumped up a level. I had been in law enforcement for nearly a decade, and all of a sudden, I was a better shooter and had better weapon-manipulation skills because my accuracy and coordination skills with the double under had improved. I learned that improving capacity in skills requiring coordination, accuracy, agility, and balance does not exist in a vacuum, and instead spreads throughout the entire body and mind, and lends improvement to any other skill requiring these same capacities.

Improving my double unders also improved my speed and skill with plyometric box jumps. I could jump down from a box and fire right back up with a much quicker reaction force.

In other words, moving the lever up on one skill can send waves throughout the systems in such a way that it's expressed in gym movements, as well as movements outside of the gym.

And when it comes to sports, there's a real payoff. Because, after you have spent time working on those general athletic skills through the kind of training outlined in this book, you have a great advantage in learning a new sport. Those general skills are hardwired into each and every sport in unique ways, and you will find that you pick up other sports swiftly.

This is one of the keys to longevity: keeping things interesting. Again, this is part of the appeal of functional-fitness conditioning. You can put it to use in having fun with different sports.

The icing on the cake is this: By learning new sports, you send new dimensions of skill through the entire system. Nuances that come with a new sport will help you make the next PR in the gym. It might even help your double unders!

One of my training partners years ago was an amazing athlete and the only person I've ever met who can do a strict one-arm pull-up with both arms. How did he get that rare skill? It came from mountain climbing!

Team sports, individual sports, outdoor activities, indoor activities—everything and anything from track to month-long sea-kayaking trips. Find a sport that intrigues you and jump in!

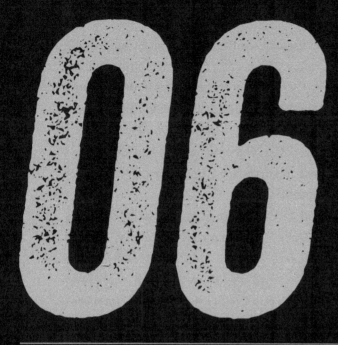

06

POWER NUTRITION

IF YOU HAD A SEVERE WEIGHT PROBLEM and walked into my gym looking for guidance, I might surprise you with my approach. I wouldn't talk about exercise or Mash-Up Threshold training or CrossFit. Not at first, anyway. The first thing I would talk about? Nutrition. In fact, I might encourage you to make that your absolute focus for a month or even several months, in addition to joining our group for hikes on the beach or trail.

When it comes to body composition, nutrition is number one. Exercise and activity are definitely important, but altering your metabolic machinery through gaining control of your nutrition is what will stimulate a radical change in body-fat levels and help you reach that weight-loss goal.

Furthermore, nutrition is not to be discarded by those who are already in good shape. Poor nutrition limits performance and recovery and increases risk of chronic disease. I tested this 16 years ago, and it's still working for me.

A sea of change has occurred in the last decade when it comes to the role of nutrition, body composition, and physical performance. The long-held belief that food is merely a calories in/calories out exchange has been replaced by a more nuanced understanding.

Here's the good news: Food is just as powerful as exercise when it comes to increasing performance, health, and longevity; burning off body fat; and increasing lean muscle tissue.

And it may even be *more* powerful. The foods we choose to eat and the portions of those foods have monumental effects on our metabolism and hormonal regulation.

What does this all mean for you? It means that the express lane to being in top physical condition is working to match your conditioning program with smart nutrition.

It's not just the express lane. It's an autobahn.

And it doesn't have to be complicated. By simply paying attention to the ratio of protein, carbs, and fats in each meal and snack, and by choosing real foods over processed foods, you'll enjoy the following benefits:

Excess body fat will become a primary energy source. Exercise will assist the process, but diet is the main driver of body composition.

Your energy levels will improve and stay consistent. If you've been eating a diet high in processed carbohydrate (for example, pasta, cereals, and breads), you'll notice this change within the first week, maybe even the first few days. Mid-afternoon low-energy crashes will vanish.

Hunger will be controlled. Reconfiguring your diet to include moderate amounts of healthy fat and protein mean less blood sugar and insulin chaos in your body. The result? You won't be under the merciless dictatorship of hunger.

Energy, stamina, and endurance in workouts will soar. A response to replacing a high-carbohydrate diet with a balanced, smart diet biased toward real foods is that the energy machinery of your body will go through a retrofit. The energy-producing mechanisms and enzymes of the cells will become more efficient at burning stored body fat. You'll notice an immediate payoff in your workouts: more power, more muscular stamina, and more cardiovascular endurance.

The diet I'm talking about is the Zone Diet, as formulated by Barry Sears, PhD, in the 1990s. Originally an MIT-trained cancer-drug researcher, Sears knew that he was genetically wired for a heart attack based on the early deaths of his father and uncles from heart disease. Sears realized that the most powerful drug, when it comes to optimal expression and repression of our genes, is not a pharmaceutical. It's food. Food can make us or ruin us. He began working with Olympic swimmers in the 1990s, and the results were clear: A diet that centered you in the sweet spot of hormonal regulation unleashed top physical performance as well as health.

My goal in this chapter is to introduce you to the basics of the diet and present you with a set of simple techniques that I used to successfully implement the diet. However, I strongly encourage you to read Sears's books to give you a deep dive into *why* food impacts our hormones the way they do.

It's been my experience as a teacher and coach that the most important task in sticking to a diet is creating a structure and routine to make it easy. Have you ever bought a diet book and felt overwhelmed by all the thinking, shopping, and cooking you'd have to do in order to follow it? In my case, I worked long, difficult shifts in law enforcement, on SWAT teams, and in the military, so making the Zone Diet easy to implement and follow was a necessity. It had to be high-speed and easy. It also had to taste good.

I'll start by introducing you to my initial experience with the Zone Diet and the "block" system that is at the heart of Sears's program. While I recommend you eventually embrace this more precise version, I'm going to finish the chapter by detailing the easiest method to begin eating in this high-powered way—a method invented by Sears that doesn't require homework or weighing food to prepare meals. It's a technique that is as effective as it is simple to do.

MY ENTRY INTO THE ZONE

I first heard about the value of implementing diet into the pursuit of high physical performance in 2002. I was attending the workouts at Coach Glassman's gym. My mind-set with those workouts, as I've mentioned, was to approach them as though my life depended on it. If I lost a workout then I could lose if things went sideways at work, too. There's a high level of unpredictability in law enforcement, and this uncertainty—the unknown and unknowable—escalates when you're dealing with a suspect who is desperate, drunk, or on drugs. So, when serving as a deputy sheriff for the Santa Cruz County Sheriff's Office, my mind-set was: I have to win in the gym. I was equating winning the workout with winning the fight for my life.

At the gym, I was part of the 6:00 a.m. crew that Coach called Team Six. The competition was fierce, and I was losing too many workouts. I went to Coach to ask how I could ramp things up.

He was talking a lot about nutrition at the time. I recall a whiteboard lecture he gave to "Team Six" where he offered his belief that the ideal way to create a "super athlete" would be to start people off by sending them to an island where for six months they would rewire their metabolism simply by eating well.

On that island, you would be thousands of miles away from soft drinks, processed food, and junk foods of all kinds. You'd be eating controlled portion sizes of a diet prepared with real foods to ensure those meals are anti-inflammatory—optimal in terms of hormonal regulation and health. After that six months of rewiring, the newly emerging athlete would have a brand-new internal foundation. And that new foundation's metabolism and hormones could then be further improved through the right kinds of physical conditioning and movement.

I wanted in on this powerful nutrition opportunity, even though there was no desert island for me to stay on. I was handed a copy of *The Zone*, a nutrition book by Sears that detailed the inner workings of the then popular (and controversial) 40/30/30 diet.

The 40/30/30 references the macronutrient ratio that Sears prescribed. It means that 40 percent of your calories should come from carbohydrate sources, 30 percent from protein, and 30 percent from fat. When Sears came out with this book in the mid-1990s, it was (no pun intended) totally against the grain. What was largely considered to be the healthiest diet was more like a 70 percent carbohydrate diet, with the balance coming from fat and protein sources.

According to Sears and Coach Glassman, if I wanted to improve my health and performance through nutrition, I needed to expand my understanding of what food was. Was food strictly a fuel source, where you took in calories and burned them? And if you didn't burn enough you'd be fat? Or, as Sears maintained, should we look at food as having an impact on our hormones, such as insulin, humane growth hormone, and testosterone?

If we look at food through the lens of its impact on the body's complex and powerful hormonal system, then it's not just how much we eat that makes a critical difference to health, energy, and performance, but what we eat and when we eat it. A diet high in carbohydrates has the potential to drive the insulin response into unhealthy areas. High carb intake also mutes the body's capacity to burn stored body fat as a ready fuel source. So when you shift your diet toward the macronutrient ratios Sears suggests, your body provides a more balanced hormonal response. And that's the prize. It means inflammation throughout the body is lower, muscle mass is higher, and body fat burns more readily.

It all sounds pretty straightforward. But, I've found that any mention of the Zone diet brings out an emotional reaction from people. There's an assumption that it's radical—that it's a super-high protein diet, something that you might see bodybuilders use.

In fact, that's not the case. "It's your grandmother's diet," Sears will tell you. It's balanced between a good helping of vegetables, a modest amount of protein, and healthy fats. I recall Coach Glassman talking about how he would run into a wall with medical doctors when he said he prescribed the

Zone Diet to his athletes. They were horrified. Then Coach would rephrase the conversation and say that a typical dinner he would advocate might include 4 to 5 ounces of chicken breast and a good helping of asparagus, perhaps drizzled in olive oil or with a tablespoon of slivered almonds. The doctor would hear this and say, "Yes! That's fantastic. That's what people should be eating." Of course, what Coach had just described was a sample Zone Diet meal.

These ideas were certainly intriguing to me—they opened my eyes in many ways—and if Coach said it was the real deal, I trusted him. After all, the radical results I was seeing from his high-intensity training using functional movements was proof enough that I should listen to him. "Tell me what to do," I said.

I was grateful to be given a five-day Zone Diet meal plan that I could implement immediately.

I bought a scale and began to weigh and measure my meals so that they fit the Zone 40/30/30 protocol. In essence, it boiled down to using the following principles:

1. Striking a key 40/30/30 balance between protein, carbohydrates, and fats at every meal.
2. Figuring out how much total protein you require each day, which means calculating the amount of lean muscle mass you have along with the amount of physical activity you do in a day.
3. Taking that protein goal for the day and distributing it among three meals and two or three snacks per day.
4. With each meal or snack, using the 40/30/30 ratio to suggest the amount of carbohydrate and fat needed to make for a balanced plate.
5. Seeking out protein sources like salmon, chicken, and lean beef and minimizing the intake of meats with high levels of saturated fats.
6. Getting most of your carbohydrate from a mix of colorful vegetables and low-sugar fruits like berries.

7. Seeking out fats of the monounsaturated variety, like olive oil, avocado, and macadamia nuts.

Before I took on this five-day program, my standard diet was high in protein with very little monounsaturated fat, and lots of pasta. Adopting the Zone program made for a big change. My protein intake came down considerably, as did my carb intake. I was also adopting a regimented structure in terms of meal timing. I would never allow five hours to pass without a snack or meal created along the 40/30/30 construct.

Portion control is a big deal with the Zone Diet. The sizes of the meals are modest. One of the values of the fat intake is that consumption of fat, along with the protein, satisfies hunger. A problem with a high-carb/low-fat diet is that this satiation is very temporary. A big plate of pasta, for example, is very high in fast-digesting carbs that spike blood sugar (the spike in blood sugar is why some foods are referred to as being "high-glycemic"). The carbs precipitate a large insulin response to store the excess blood sugar. Oddly enough, this leads to being hungry in a very short time, despite the meal.

As portions, I was allotted 22 blocks of food a day for my size and exercise level—five four-block meals and a two-block snack. According to the Zone, average men and women need 14 and 11 blocks per day, respectively; a 6-foot, 185-pound man would use 16 or 17 blocks. I was allotted the extra blocks based on my high activity level and my body weight at that time, which was a lean 200 pounds. (The protein requirement in the Zone Diet hinges on how much lean muscle mass you have. The more lean muscle mass, the more protein required. Volume and intensity of activity also elevates the number of protein blocks required.)

A block, under the Zone system, is a balanced unit of food, composed of the following three sub-blocks that apply to all, regardless of activity level, body composition, or age:

PROTEIN	7 grams	i.e., one ounce of chicken, turkey, or sardines; two ounces of shrimp or two egg whites; high-fat meats like bacon, sausage, hot dogs, marbled meats, and duck aren't ideal. Go for leaner meats and cuts.
CARB	9 grams	i.e., half an apple, four cups of broccoli, a quarter-cup of black beans; not recommended are carbs from processed grains, like bread or pasta.
FAT	1.5 grams	i.e., three olives, three almonds, or a teaspoon of olive oil.

Barry Sears has worked with a number of world-class athletes. An athlete eating a Zone Diet correctly calibrated to his or her lean muscle mass and physical activity who is still hungry will want to first dial up the macronutrient of fat. In my case, I immediately doubled the fat intake in my Zone experiment.

That's an important detail to underscore: Dr. Sears advises athletes to double the fat intake if they are already at an ideal leanness with their body composition. That was my case: I was in very good condition and training extremely hard. If I hadn't been exercising so hard, or if I had an excess amount of fat to lose, I would not have doubled the fat intake per the Zone protocol. So bear this in mind as I describe what I did. Eating 24 almonds within a meal was how I achieved the high-fat intake I was prescribed.

For a month I measured and prepped each meal, using a food scale to be precise. I continued training and logging workout results in my journal, curious to see what would happen. It didn't take long for me to begin registering considerable gains. I started taking 10 seconds to 2 minutes off certain benchmark workouts and showing tremendous gains in power output and stamina. Additionally, my personal records for the deadlift, squat, and press went up by 10 pounds or more each.

I also noticed improvements in my well-being and cognitive performance. I was sharper mentally and I felt a more consistent balance of emotional energy. Given the stress of my daily job, these positive effects were invaluable.

The challenge that I faced was one that anyone on any diet faces: building it into my day. I had to make it work for a job where I was often on patrol. How could I consume a 22-block Zone Diet throughout a workday? I quickly discovered the answer: precooking meals and Tupperware.

It looked like this:

BREAKFAST (MEAL #1) 4 blocks

PROTEIN	4 scrambled eggs	4 blocks of protein
CARB	1⅓ cup oatmeal	⅓ cup oatmeal is 1 block
FAT	24 almonds	for 8 blocks (an example of 2× the fat intake)

LUNCH (MEAL #2) 4 blocks

PROTEIN	1 cup cottage cheese	¼ cup per block, equalling 4 blocks of protein
CARB	2 apples sliced into the cottage cheese	half an apple is 1 block
FAT	24 almonds	again, 2× the fat; this equals 8 blocks of fat, as 3 almonds make 1 block of fat

MEAL #3 4 blocks

PROTEIN	4 ounces lean red meat, usually a flank steak sliced very thin	4 blocks of protein
CARB	1 cup spaghetti with the meat stirred into the pasta	4 blocks of carbohydrate
FAT	2 tablespoons of olive oil	2× the fat—⅓ teaspoon olive oil equals 1 block of fat

MEAL #4	4 blocks	
PROTEIN	4 ounces sliced cheese	4 blocks of protein
CARB	1 Fuji apple sliced thin and 1 cup blueberries	4 blocks of carbohydrate
FAT	24 almonds	8 blocks of fat

At this point in the day, I had consumed a total of 18 blocks of food. This left me with 4 blocks to eat when I headed home after work for dinner. I always tried to make a meal heavy in vegetables as the source of carbohydrate. I made up any shortage in carbohydrate blocks with Fuji apples.

DINNER (MEAL #5)	4 blocks	
PROTEIN	4 ounces lean meat or fish	4 blocks of protein
CARB	large salad with broccoli, tomatoes, spinach, and cucumber	4 blocks of carbohydrate
FAT	24 almonds	8 blocks of fat

Occasionally I worked overtime, and I had to be prepared for those meals. My solution was to drop into a grocery or convenience store and purchase string cheese (protein) and an apple (carb). I also always carried extra almonds (fat) with me.

Water is the drink of choice in the Zone Diet. I applied the weight-and-measure doctrine to this as well, drinking from a one-gallon container, making sure I got 64 ounces of water per day at minimum.

Since February 2002, this is the method that I've used to eat. Pretty simple, right? There have been times I've calibrated the fat intake to match an increase in training intensity and volume. Another alteration I began experimenting with was to upgrade the total quality of my carbohydrate intake, trimming out any carbs that I was getting from processed foods like pasta and making sure I was getting all of my carbs from vegetables and fruits. It was a powerful modification: I lost five more pounds of body fat from this simple change, even while consuming as much as four times the fat of the traditional Zone protocol.

I want to emphasize that I am not a doctor or nutritionist. Rather, I am simply a very experienced coach and athlete who has been following the Zone Diet for more than 15 years—and teaching it to others. If you and I were talking, and you told me you have special medical concerns or dietary restrictions, I would certainly suggest you work with your doctor for help in dialing in your diet with routine blood work to take some of the guesswork out of the process.

I also encourage you to read one or more of Sears's books. Two helpful ones, which also include recipes, are *Enter the Zone* and *Mastering the Zone*. They explain in more detail how the diet works, how to calculate your protein needs for the day, and how to calculate your blocks. I also recommend two other titles, *Zone Food Blocks* and *Zone Perfect Meals in Minutes*, to help you make the transition to the high-end of the diet as easy as possible. Additionally, visit my website www.firebreatherfitness.org for videos and articles on how I teach and approach the Zone Diet.

HOW TO GET STARTED NOW

The simplest way to begin eating Zone-based meals is to use the Eyeball Method that Sears teaches. It's not as precise as the block method, but it will get you very close to the sweet spot.

First, commit to eating three meals each day with two or three Zone snacks.

Next, build your meals like so: Set out a dinner plate. Mentally divide it into thirds.

Fill one-third of the plate with a healthy protein source, such as chicken, lean beef, fish, or turkey. It should amount to about what would fit in the palm of your hand.

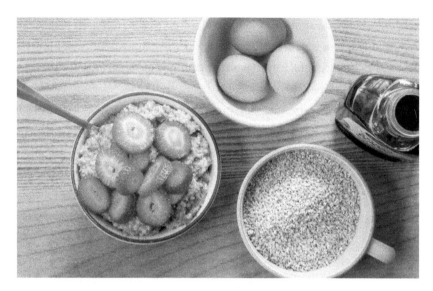

AMUNDSON'S OATMEAL

Put 2 cups of water into a saucepan and bring to a boil. Add 1 teaspoon of salt, then add 1 cup of quick-cooking steel-cut oats. Cover and simmer 7 to 10 minutes. Remove from heat. Add 1 tablespoon of butter, a teaspoon of cinnamon, and a hint of agave nectar, and stir. One cup of cooked oatmeal is 3 blocks of carbohydrate. Eat with 3 hard-boiled eggs for the 3 blocks of protein. This results in a perfect 3-block meal.

Fill the remaining two-thirds of the dinner plate with vegetables and fruits as your carbs. Opt mostly for different colored vegetables. With fruits, lean toward berries, which are high in nutrients and relatively low in sugar. If you choose a processed carb instead, like rice or potatoes, reduce the amount to about the same size as your protein source.

Finally, add a healthy fat. Salad dressing (like a vinaigrette with olive oil and vinegar), a slice of avocado or macadamia nuts (1 macadamia nut equals 1 fat block), or almonds (3 almonds equal 1 fat block) are ideal.

And that's it. Each of your meals should fit this description. Between meals, or before a workout, have a snack. String cheese and an apple is an example of a Zone-favorable snack. To devise one, think in terms of a small portion of protein balanced by a carbohydrate, plus a dose of built-in fat. Examples include an ounce of turkey, ½ an apple, and a few nuts, or a hard-boiled egg, a handful of berries, and a slice of avocado. Simple selections.

Other ideas for snacks include:

SNACK #1 2 blocks

5 strawberries, chopped
½ cup blueberries
6 almonds

put it all on top of:
½ cup cottage cheese
Stevia to taste

SNACK #2 1 block

1 oz. low-fat string cheese
1 kiwi
1 tbsp. peanut butter

SNACK #3 2 blocks

2 oz. chicken breast
1 Fuji apple, sliced
6 almonds

MIND

07

HARNESSING THE POWER OF YOUR MIND

AS YOU RAISE THE INTENSITY LEVELS of your Firebreather workouts, the importance of mental strength becomes increasingly apparent. The greater the discomfort you can produce in a workout, the greater its potency and the more you'll progress. But here's the catch: the harder the workout, the more of a role the mind will play. This equation applies not only to physical exercise and training but also to the many challenges we set for ourselves and those we face in life in general.

The pursuit of a career on a law-enforcement SWAT team, or as a member of a military special operations unit, certainly presents intense challenges. In the selection and assessment process of the United States's most elite units, it's hard to tell which recruits will, by the end of the process, make the final cut. The vast majority of candidates who start the process do not finish. But surprisingly, after torturous crucibles like Navy SEAL BUD/S training, including Hell Week, during which candidates face nonstop physical and psychological torment without sleep for five days, it's not necessarily the physically fittest who make it. In fact, it's some of the "best" athletes at the start of the process who are the first to drop out. Although it varies from class to class, of the few who do qualify to enter BUD/S, the dropout rate is typically high; as many as one in four who begin the program quit.

What is at work for those who succeed? In physically challenging environments, both in the gym and in life, those who survive—and even thrive—often demonstrate a strong sense of purpose and use a basic set of mental tools and stress-control techniques.

In physically challenging environments, those who survive— and even thrive—often demonstrate a strong sense of purpose and use a basic set of mental tools and stress-control techniques.

In fact, in the years following 9/11 when the demand for Navy SEAL units intensified, the Navy Special Warfare Command began to look at how to improve the screening process, and brought on Eric Potterat, PhD, a clinical sports psychologist who took on the role of teaching skills to improve performance in active-duty SEALs as well as prepare applicants to have a better shot of making it through training. Although Potterat, a scientist, is hesitant to state that the implementation of sports psychology is directly responsible for improving resiliency and performance in SEALs and want-to-be SEALs, he did say on a law-enforcement podcast the following: "The BUD/S rates [of success] have gotten better. The research supports that our resilience in the community is strong."

In his work with the SEALs in Coronado, California, Potterat took advantage of the strong relationship the Navy has with the nearby US Olympic Training Center in Chula Vista. A resident psychologist there offered a quote that Potterat feels is as applicable to world-class athletes as it is to those who succeeded at BUD/S and those who failed: "The difference between a gold medal and no medal is all between the ears."

I couldn't agree more.

The skills that Potterat believes are essential revolve around the following: managing stress through breathing techniques, positive self-talk, and focus and concentration during training. Successful candidates also tend to manage their challenges in several key ways:

» By setting incremental goals.
» By managing their mental state by dismissing negative thoughts and harboring positive ones.
» By working to control fear, worry, and stress over what can't be controlled and redirecting this into energy and effort aimed at what can be controlled.
» By focusing on the process, the day-in and day-out training, without rigid attachment to the results.
» By discerning what is temporary and what is permanent.
» By disciplining internal dialogue and self-talk.
» By breaking down large goals into incremental, bite-size pieces.

Combined, these skills allow the successful candidates to use unhindered mental power. The same positive flow can apply for you. Hone the above skills, endeavor to apply them consistently day after day, and turn them into habits. Do that, and you will discover that tough goals become not barriers but rather kindling for the fire, a fire that will allow you to attack an even wider range of goals than those that once might have paralyzed you with fear.

Let's look at a real-life challenge. Say your goal is to lose 10 pounds. Achieving this objective requires some very simple changes: establish better eating habits, cut down (or cut out) beer, sleep better, and exercise consistently. Nothing magical there! It's common sense.

It really is that simple. But is it easy? That depends upon your mental approach to the goal, and to the tasks and routines you put in place around it. Those same key areas that allow some candidates to triumph in their pursuit of joining the special operations community (such as purpose, goal-setting, self-talk, and managing fear and stress) will play incredibly potent roles in your success.

The scenario that often plays out is all too common. It may have even happened to you—times that you've started with a goal but soon gave up on trying to make changes.

You begin with a desire to look and feel better. In order to do so, you set out to lose those 10 pounds. But outside of a hazy desire of wanting to lose the weight, there's no focused thinking about it or pursuit of information on how best to make it happen. There's no direct application of skills to override the current programming of poor habits. The mind instead sinks into memories of perhaps having failed at earlier attempts to adopt a diet and exercise program. Those thoughts—embroiled with fear of failing—soon translate into a sense of giving up and giving in. "I'll never be able to do it" or "I hate myself for being so weak" are the types of vulture-like judgments circling in your mind. Thoughts lead to choices and actions, and these sorts of negative thoughts lead to sinking into the couch and self-medicating with beer, pizza, ice cream, or binge television.

Which leads to the opposite of the results you truly desire!

But this is not a no-win or inevitable situation. Not by a long shot. Consistently applying simple actions and skills, harnessing the power of your mind, focusing on key areas, and honing the mental tools that serve these areas will lead to the positive results you are seeking.

The first step is finding and articulating purpose. What do you want? What do you stand for? Why are you here and what are you going to do about it?

THE POWER OF POSITIVE TENSE

In the spring of 2011, I was doing a phone consultation with an athlete who was a contender to win that year's CrossFit Games. He had been working tirelessly on achieving a freestanding handstand push-up, with little success. Frustrated, he thought for sure that in order to achieve that goal, he needed physical technique coaching. Hearing the anxiety in his voice, I asked, "Brother, tell me in your own words what you are trying to achieve. What exactly is your goal?"

He responded, "I'm trying to do a freestanding handstand push-up without falling over."

I replied, "Brother, that's not what you really want. What you really want to do is a freestanding handstand push-up while maintaining your balance."

The conversation got very silent, and finally he said, "I'll call you back."

The very next day, the athlete called me and happily announced he had achieved his goal.

What had changed?

He simply changed an internal message that had been imprinted on his mind. Before our conversation, the message he'd been playing over and over had actually resulted in him falling over, although this is not what he had wanted. Imprinting the positive tense helped him communicate to his subconscious mind what he really wanted, and not the opposite of it.

Change the message, change your world.

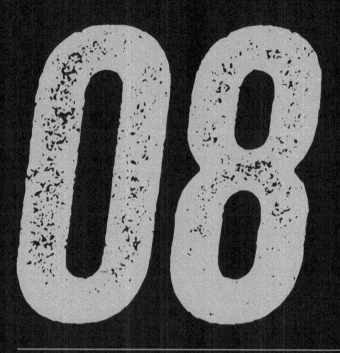

08

FINDING YOUR PURPOSE

IN THE SUMMER OF 2012, I shared a stage with Kyle Maynard, a world-renowned public speaker on topics of personal motivation, leadership, and developing a strong sense of life purpose. Kyle is unstoppable when it comes to his own purpose, that of inspiring others. Among his many achievements, including winning 36 wrestling matches in high school, Kyle became a mixed-martial artist despite being born without arms and legs. He put his life story into his supercharged book, *No Excuses*. More recently, the ESPY-award-winner climbed Mount Kilimanjaro without the aid of prosthetics.

Kyle and I were both speakers at the Adaptive Athlete Wounded Warrior Summit in Texas, and Kyle stole the show with a captivating life lesson about overcoming obstacles and overwhelming odds.

Kyle proposes that the majority of people spend their life existing mainly in the "what" circle of existence. They use all of their life energy and willpower responding to what is happening in their life, never stopping to consider their own responsibility in what is occurring, and more impor-tantly, that they have the power to change their future situations by taking leadership of their life. Some break through to the next circle, the "how." For them, instead of worrying about "what" is happening, they focus on "how" they can make mindful choices that affect their future conditions and experiences. Only a very few people ever make the leap into the "why" circle, Kyle says. This is the most profound place to live, because from this circle, we begin to contemplate not merely "what" or "how" but rather "why" life is unfolding as it is. This question ultimately leads one to con-sider the biggest questions, such as, "why was I born?," "why do I behave in this manner?," and "what is my purpose here?" It's the pursuit of answers to these questions that leads to a meaningful and fulfilling life. The key, Kyle explains, is to continually move the direction of your life closer to the "why." Kyle says that when we attach a strong and compelling "why" to a goal, our staying power and strength of will is immensely increased.

After Kyle's presentation, we had an opportunity to compare notes. Kyle said something to me that day that I will always remember: "Greg, the stronger the why in your life, the stronger your life will be."

To successfully tackle the challenges of the Firebreather Fitness pro-gram, it is important for you to have a strong sense of purpose, and a com-pelling reason "why" you are going to commit to the training, day in and day out. In the warrior professions of military service and law enforce-ment, I have often said, "train as if your life depends on it—because it does." What could be a more compelling reason for a law-enforcement officer or military operator to train than the cold hard truth that their level of readiness could easily mean the difference between life and death? That certainly helped focus and fuel my own purpose and commitment. What about yours? What is your why?

Your purpose in life is unique to you, and your talents, skills, and attri-butes allow you to fulfill that purpose in your unique way. A purpose and a goal are not the same things, although they are related. (Goals will be dis-cussed in greater detail in Chapter 9.) Think of purpose as the goalposts

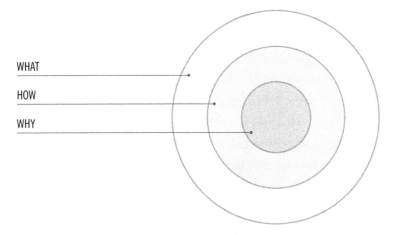

WHAT

HOW

WHY

The "What-How-Why" concept was introduced to me by Kyle Maynard during the 2012 Wounded Warrior Summit in Austin, Texas. Kyle was the keynote speaker at the event, which teaches leadership, positive life strategies, and the warrior mind-set to soldiers and marines who have suffered catastrophic injuries in combat.

on a football field, whereas goals are the plays that move the ball down the field. Your purpose is the "why" of your life. When you become clear on your purpose, the choices you make either move you closer to the goalposts, or farther away. However, until you awaken to the purpose of your life, it will be hard to determine which way you are moving the ball. In fact, you could easily end up moving backward.

Having a strong sense of "why" is essential when it comes to developing and maintaining any physical discipline, especially a challenging fitness plan such as Firebreather Fitness. Because it doesn't get easier. As you progress into the program and your strength, stamina, endurance, and all-around fitness increase, you will find out what I found out: As you get fitter, the work gets harder! It demands more from you—more mental strength and more discipline to push through the discomfort of the daily sessions as you pursue your goals. I was able to make consistent progress in my training for more than 15 years. But that demanded that I invest in the "why" of my training in order to be able to show up for a workout day in, day out, year after year. Without that investment, enthusiasm and focus melt away and it is all too easy to drift away from the program. With that investment, however, you become excited to show up each day to do the work, with that same excitement that you had on Day One.

In addition, when you land on the *why* of your training, a powerful shift in awareness takes place. That awareness helps you to more clearly discern where, when, and how to apply your willpower in the achievement of your goals. For example, in a competitive workout, it's easy to focus on other people and their performances. But splitting your attention between your effort and the effort of others is like splitting your own strength in half, using one portion of your potential. When you instead focus your mind upon what you can influence, you increase your potential.

So here's the upshot: Developing and harnessing your full mental power begins with selecting and defining your purpose. Purpose is your supreme power source. A weak or vague sense of purpose is like drawing a bow halfway. Your purpose needs to be fully drawn, tapping into your deepest passions and values. It is more than just a goal, reaching above and beyond, say, doing 20 pull-ups or having a six-pack. There is nothing wrong with those physical goals; however, your purpose should get at something bigger. It should take you into a territory where you'd put your life on the line to fight for it. If you don't know your purpose, your why, then you diminish your chance of successfully achieving your goals. You will almost certainly fall short of your full potential.

FINDING YOUR FIREPOWER

Purpose is a very personal thing. Yours may be wrapped around being a parent, or a teacher, or a coach, or owning a successful business, or pursuing a career you dream about.

If your purpose serves as your goalposts, then you want every play to move the football down the field, closer to those posts. Over the course of your life, however, your purpose may evolve. For example, in my early twenties, I identified my purpose as "to protect and serve my community

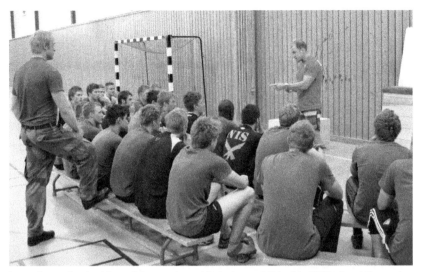

Lecturing on leadership and the warrior spirit during a visit to the 137th Royal Norwegian Air Force Military Police Unit.

as a law-enforcement officer." After three years of serving as a deputy sheriff, however, I knew I wanted to serve and protect in a greater capacity, and thus my purpose expanded as well. "I want to protect and serve my community, and my country, by serving as a warrior in the military and law enforcement." My redefined purpose ultimately led me into the Army and Drug Enforcement Administration. As I continued to mature and learn more about my unique talents and passions, I began to feel strongly that my purpose had more to do with educating and inspiring the warrior professions to pursue holistic fitness. As a result, my purpose was refined once again.

All along my path toward becoming a Firebreather, it was this purpose that fueled my dedication to hard physical training. The fuel source was especially plentiful in law enforcement and the military, of course. Lives were on the line, including my own, so the quality of my workouts had a life-or-death edge to them. I had no shortage of energy to use toward pushing myself through punishing workouts and making sacrifices to remain committed to my purpose.

That is where your fitness program comes in. No matter what your purpose is, I truly believe it can be best supported and expressed by the development of a strong mind, body, and spirit. Therefore, dedication to a fitness program is critical to achieving not only a variety of goals but also the very purpose of your life. After all, at the end of the day, it's all one, integrated whole that we're talking about: body, mind, and spirit. Everything has to be in alignment in order for you to be at your peak potential. Serving and giving your all toward a great life purpose will not be fulfilled without basic daily disciplines to improve your body, mind, and spirit.

Indeed, the firepower in being a Firebreather comes directly from purpose, and the work to uncover and develop yours is a necessary starting point to getting the most out of your physical workouts.

If you don't feel like you have a strong purpose right now, or you feel like the path you're currently on is not in tune with a deep-down sense of what you feel you were born to do, now is a great time to begin listening to the signals that will lead you toward one of the most important revelations in your life.

Realizing your purpose is more than just a conscious act. Your purpose resides in the subconscious, spiritual realm. To access this inner stream requires creating a space of silence in the judgmental, critical part of the mind instead of drowning it out with the usual noise, doubts, or lures from, say, messages being transmitted by the many marketing forces trying to capture your interest 24/7.

Your tools for creating the quiet you need to discover your purpose are many: meditation, long walks in nature, solitude, prayer, and freewriting in a journal are all great avenues. The aim is to dwell in a place where images and messages from your own inner stream can bubble to the surface.

To begin, the questions you plant are simple ones: What do I truly want? What do I stand for? Why am I here and what am I going to do about it?

These are simple questions, but they're big ones, and at first you may have a hard time answering them.

Plant your questions through meditation, prayer, or journal writing—whatever works for you—and then listen deeply. Be patient and pay attention. Give your best to this process, and you will be rewarded with deep insights about who you are and what you are here to do.

You'll know you're moving in the right direction in identifying your purpose when the answers to your questions require from you things such as sacrifice, discomfort, hard work, setbacks, pain, risk, and failures along the way. But I promise, this is the good stuff! It forges a path that leads toward inner knowledge, cornering you into plumbing the depths of your soul for courage and strength.

I can't tell you exactly how long this process will take. Some discover their purpose and passion early on. Others don't find it until later in life. For some the process is prompted by a severe jolt to their life—perhaps the loss of a loved one or a near-death experience. Others simply are struck by the knowledge that they are ready for change, ready for more, ready to embrace all they can be.

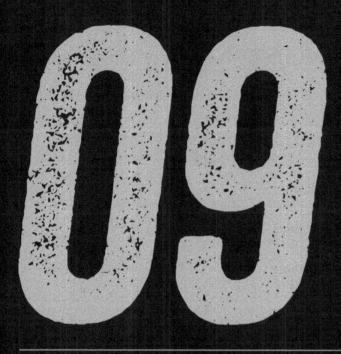

09

SETTING AND REACHING YOUR GOALS

WHILE FINDING OR REFINING YOUR PURPOSE is a nonlinear, spiritual process, creating a structure of smartly written goals that will enable you to wisely invest your time and work efforts is a far more mechanical process, one well worth your careful thought and attention. Setting smart, sound goals will not only help you stay on track but will also funnel your attention to the present moment—ultimately the most valuable resource you have when you're turning goals into realities.

As you consider your goals, think big. Goals should provide you with motivation, inspiration, and direction. Goals should fire you up! They should make you jump out of bed in the morning, and make you want to devote your free time to them. Whereas your purpose is your defining principle for being here—whether it's as down-to-earth and profound as being a good parent, or as lofty as dedicating your life to finding a cure for cancer—your goals are the clear-cut, defined objectives that pave the pursuit of that purpose.

These big goals can be broken down into smaller, incremental goals, which are so important that I will discuss them in greater detail shortly. In brief, they are derived from the major goals in your life. Your big goals are like the rooftop you want to ascend to, with incremental, tangible, immediate goals like the rungs on a ladder you are climbing to get up there.

The very first step in goal-setting for the Firebreather Fitness program is to understand and define the word "goal" within the context of athleticism and personal achievement. Inspired by years of mentoring athletes aiming to achieve their dreams, I have created a definition that includes three important points of performance:

Goal: A specifically desired end state, expressed in the positive tense and set within a realistic time frame, that provides motivation and direction on the path to achievement. Let's examine that definition a little bit closer. I want to expand upon those three points of performance.

1. **The goal must be specific.** For example, "I want to complete 50 consecutive gymnastic kipping pull-ups." The more focused the definition, the more opportunity there is for precise planning, preparation, and training. In addition, by specifically defining a goal, an athlete can evaluate with precision when the goal has been met.

2. **The goal is best expressed in the positive tense, stating what you want, not what you don't want.** For example, "I want $10,000" is positive tense. "I don't want to be in debt" is negative tense. Think in terms of plenty, not lack.

There is great power in stating goals positively. If I say to myself, "I don't want to fall off the climbing rope," the image of falling is central to the statement. This image can create fear and further propel the image, almost as if I'd thought, "I want to fall off the climbing rope." By telling yourself what you don't want to manifest, you create a blueprint for exactly what you intend to avoid. The key lesson for athletes is to keep the mind in a state of positive affirmation of the goal's desired outcome.

3. **The goal must include a time frame that is challenging yet realistic and achievable.** A goal set too far in the future will lack urgency and fail to create the internal fire needed for accomplishment. On the other hand, too short a time frame can lead to discouragement and despair. In setting a time frame for a goal, you must weigh the delicate balance between motivating and challenging yourself while at the same time ensuring a high likelihood of success.

When deciding upon the time frame, some self-assessment is required. For example, if an athlete told me his goal is to perform a single set of 50 pull-ups in three months, I would ask how many consecutive pull-ups he can currently complete. How specifically the athlete can answer that question will help me determine the best approach to supporting his achievement of the goal. If the athlete does not know how many pull-ups he can do right now, we need to find out! The approach we take to setting a time frame for completing 50 consecutive pull-ups will vary greatly if the athlete has five pull-ups as compared with 45 pull-ups.

Once a goal is set, it is helpful to "see" it. Use drawings, magazine images, and visualizations. Our mind thinks in pictures, so it is important to imprint upon your mind a detailed image of what you want to achieve. You should also assign an emotion to your goal. Imagine how you will feel when your goal is accomplished. This attachment will help you push toward your goal.

So you've got a big goal—that's fantastic! The next question is—how will you get there?

MICROGOALS—RUNGS ON A LADDER

Big goals are critical. Along with purpose, they are your power source for the daily work you must invest to bring those goals to fruition.

Because of their weight and magnitude, however, big goals can be so awe-inspiring that they are overwhelming. From your starting point, the road toward their achievement can look so impossibly difficult that you may feel anxious, find it hard to start, or be tempted to quit.

Consider a woman running her first marathon. She has a background of jogging a couple of miles a few times a week. In setting a goal of running a marathon, she may find that fear of the unknown and fear of failure can be daunting if her mind tries to come to terms with all of the work required. When considered all at once, the workload necessary to transform body, mind, and spirit into a being that can run 26.2 consecutive miles can suddenly feel overwhelming.

A marathon is one example, but there are many. A college student decides he wants to become a medical doctor, in line with his purpose in life of wanting to help people. But the road toward becoming a physician takes many years of hard, intense work and sacrifice. If he thinks about this decade-plus-long journey all at a single time, fear and anxiety may poison him, making him miserable, disrupting sleep, and exhausting him before the first step.

Whether it's building a bridge, building a career, becoming a SWAT operator, creating a successful business from scratch, finishing a marathon, or becoming a full-blown Firebreather, the "killer app" skill is no doubt the skill of setting microgoals. Also called segmenting, setting microgoals pulls you back from the brink of being overwrought by a massive goal. When you stumble into thinking of the whole project all at once, and the blood pressure ticks upward, retraining your focal point to a single, simple step forward is crucial.

Andy Stumpf is a former Navy SEAL instructor who became interested in why candidates who had dreamt of becoming SEALs their entire lives gave in to quitting in the early stages of BUD/S. Most of those who drop out during the infamous Hell Week do so in the first day or two. Andy watched this as an instructor, with the added perspective of once being a candidate himself.

The answer soon became clear to him: Many of those who dropped out thought of Hell Week as being a one-week test that they had to get through in order to become a SEAL. When it's 4 a.m., five hours after Hell Week has begun, the scale of five days of unending punishment with no sleep is way too much to picture. In the face of that magnitude of work, some lost resolve and quit.

What of those who were able to grind their way through? They used a form of tunnel vision to refrain from worrying about making it through the entire week. Rather, they narrowed their focus on a single objective within their immediate grasp. They worked to make it through the next hour, for example. Andy says that he used microgoals when he went through Hell Week himself, thinking only about making it to the next meal and blocking out the rest. He concentrated his energy toward the single objective of making it through all of the drills and surf torture, running and exercise, just long enough to get to lunch. This was his "rung on the ladder." Once there, he would reset his vision toward making it to dinner. Then, nothing else in the universe mattered to serving his purpose except for staying in the game until breakfast. Step by step by step, this use of microgoals allowed him to keep his mind in a place where the goals could be comprehended and dealt with.

As your Firebreather workouts gain in intensity and difficulty, they become excellent opportunities to practice microgoals. A 15-minute workout in my program will be—and should be—intense. Now, on the one hand, a person could approach that workout in muddling fashion, lifting some weights here and there, avoiding focus or urgency. It may not feel quite as hard in that case, true. The 15 minutes might pass painlessly, and quickly. But the "reward" will be a disappointing lack of results.

However, Firebreather workouts are designed to ensure that they have a strong sense of focus and urgency to them. A quarter of an hour takes on a whole different meaning when you're giving your all. For example, giving your best effort in an AMRAP (as many rounds as possible) of push-ups and kettlebell swings is going to be tough. An AMRAP requires intent, focus, courage, and a purpose strong enough to sustain the effort through the waves of increasing discomfort. You'll sweat, suffer, and be forced to confront negative thoughts and maybe a desire to quit early.

Once you make it through, however, the rewards are profound. Physically, you'll make optimal gains. Mentally, you'll have more confidence. It will have been time spent as a Firebreather, solidifying your new path forward.

The toughness and intensity of these workouts makes setting microgoals crucial. They are the key to embracing the discomfort and intensity of a workout, in order to yield its benefits and move closer to your big goal. Don't think of the workout as a 15-minute whole. Rather, break it up. One way to break it up is in three 5-minute periods. Begin the workout with your total focus on the first five minutes only. Once that's conquered, turn all of your attention to the next five minutes. If the discomfort is rising quickly, you can adjust this to one minute at a time. Or perhaps to a single round of push-ups and kettlebell swings. Or, you might break up each round with five breaths. So after finishing a round, put the kettlebell down, count five breaths, then begin the next round, focused solely on finishing the new round. Climb one step up the ladder at a time.

When you practice the microgoal technique, you'll be surprised at how much ground you cover thinking in segments. Psychologically, the workout will feel faster.

Outside the gym, this technique of microgoals can be used in other aspects of your life as far as serving your greater purpose. The key elements are narrowing the focus to a specific segment of activity to accomplish, blocking everything else out of your mind, and adding deadline pressure to the task. Then when you finish that task, you put your eyes, heart, and mind on the next incremental task.

Let's revisit our marathoner. Microgoals got her through those long weeks of training. Now, as the race unfolds, she may well find it useful to employ this technique again. When she hits the 20-mile mark, she faces a final 6 miles that are a great deal different than the first 6. While the first 20 miles might have been easily broken into 5-mile segments, the last 6—where discomfort climbs hard and fast—may require thinking in terms of a mile at a time. Or a half-mile at a time. Or holding a pace to the next aid station or lamppost, then recalibrating.

In another example, let's say you have a goal of 15 strict pull-ups, and that you can currently do 5 (this number could be lower or higher, depending on your own fitness and background). How will you close that gap? First set a realistic time frame. A 6-week plan might be appropriate, involving completing two 21-day cycles of Firebreather Fitness training, and then supplementing that by performing an additional session of pull-ups each day, starting with 5 and building to 15, in incremental sets. Along the way, don't forget to visualize yourself completing 15 consecutive strict pull-ups.

Now that you have a goal and a broad plan of how to get there, you can break it down further, jotting down the small, incremental steps that can be accomplished immediately. Your list of microgoals for Day One might be:

» Perform the day's Firebreather Fitness workout.
» After the workout, complete 5 pull-ups in as few sets as possible.
» Spend five minutes visualizing yourself completing 15 consecutive pull-ups.

And so on. In sum, clarify a road map of goals that serve your purpose. Break those goals down into more immediate objectives by creating a list of bite-sized microgoals. Then go after these one by one.

When they're broken down into pieces and you put all of your focus into executing these pieces one at a time, you prevent yourself from allowing your mind to drift toward being intimidated by the big-picture goals you've set for yourself, goals that sometimes take months and years of daily toil.

Microgoals bring your dreams into the present. Sure, this means you are working toward their realization one inch at a time, but this is the best way to actualize your ambitions! The most effective way to make your dreams a reality is to break them down into microgoals, get the first one done, and then focus on the second one. This is the secret to big success.

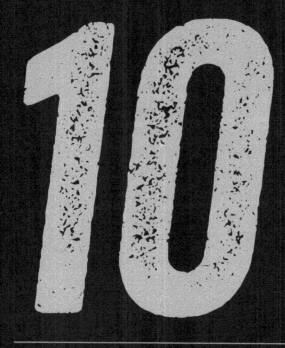

10

SELF-TALK

SELF-TALK IS ANOTHER POWERFUL TOOL to help move you on a steady and productive ascent toward your long-term goals. It is especially important when the course gets challenging, which a Firebreather path is bound to do at some points along the way.

Timothy Noakes, MD, a renowned sports scientist and author, is largely credited with a theory called the "central governor." It looks at the neurobiology of the brain's wiring in regard to discomfort and pain when we push into extremes of exercise. The brain's mechanisms are such that discomfort can be extraordinarily high even though there are still reserves of energy in the muscles. It's as if once you get below a quarter of the gas tank, a computer in the car starts forcing the engine to slow down and even stop. It's a self-protective mechanism.

In regard to getting a top endurance performance out of the body when engaged in a difficult competition, Noakes believes that the minute we allow a thought to slip into the internal dialogue—like "I'm not sure

I can do this," or "I can't keep this up," or "I think I'm going to lose"—the brain chemistry catches wind of this and immediately begins to increase the level of discomfort. Holding the pace or intensity of the effort instantly gets harder.

If we revisit our example of a first-time marathoner from Chapter 9, you can imagine what Noakes is describing taking effect. Because the athlete has never run 26 miles before, self-doubt is lurking and may take advantage of the situation if given the opportunity. There's pain, fatigue, cramping muscles, and a long way to go. As thoughts begin to circle in her head, thoughts like "I don't think I can keep going," then, per Noakes's model, things start caving in. The legs feel heavier. The discomfort grows. More negative thoughts flow. Quitting becomes more likely.

Taking control of the thoughts you're feeding your mind is invaluable. Negative thoughts and images of failure make everything heavier and harder. Positive thoughts have the opposite effect on the brain. They increase self-confidence, motivation, and personal success.

Don't be afraid to literally shout out in the middle of a workout, "Yes, I can do it!"

Do you doubt that the nature of our thoughts can be that powerful? An example from my own past illuminates this principle well.

When I was in the 41st consecutive hour of all-out physical exertion at Kokoro Camp, I found myself struggling with a task of carrying a heavy stone for a matter of hours. Instructor Mark Divine saw that I was losing ground and came over to help me get my mind right. It was a heavy rock to begin with, and my negative self-talk was making the rock feel much heavier.

As I struggled with the rock, Mark asked me, "What dog are you feeding?" Mark coaches the principle of positive self-talk using the metaphor of feeding a dog. As Mark puts it, at any given moment your thoughts are likely either feeding the dog of courage or the dog of fear. Thoughts of defeat or worry feed the dog of fear. Feed the dog of fear and he gets stronger, making things worse and increasing the chance that you'll give up. However, when you feed the dog of courage, the opposite effect takes place. You feel stronger, more certain of yourself, and cultivate an increased sense of personal belief. Feed the dog of courage with thoughts like, "I've got this!" or thoughts that focus you on making it to the next microgoal. Feeding the courage dog keeps your life energy flowing in the direction you want to go.

When it comes to the more intense workouts in your Firebreather Fitness plan, how do you starve the dog of fear and feed the dog of courage? Try this simple step-by-step process:

1. As a workout grows in intensity, be aware as thoughts emerge. Identify and acknowledge these thoughts as small pieces of food that will feed one of the internal dogs.
2. If it's a negative thought, stop it in its tracks. Calmly put it to a halt. Be sure you're not holding your breath—let breathing move in and out smoothly.
3. Perform a redirect. Let go of the negative thought and manage the energy. Redirect the negative emotional energy into a positive image or statement. Use positive statements and jingles as bits of food to feed the courage dog. Be aware of how this translates to energy and power output to be used toward the attainment of the current goal.

What would this process look like for me at that moment in Kokoro Camp? There I was, sleep-deprived, soaked head to socks from crossing a chilly stretch of salt water, exhausted, and under pressure to get back to the base in a certain amount of time, all while hauling a heavy rock. It's not hard to imagine a negative thought bubbling up like, "I don't think I can do this." My first task in this case was to be in a state of awareness so as to catch the thought early, like using a net to snare a poisonous moth. Then, in place of that thought, I could insert one with a positive emotional charge to it: I've got this! I'm doing this!

My job was to repeat these positive thoughts one after the other, feeding the courage dog and building an internal momentum toward my goal.

This technique has applications toward all sorts of challenging projects and situations, from lengthy or intense workouts to running a marathon, to studying for finals to preparing for an interview. Monitor your thoughts, feed your courage, and starve your fear.

Don't be afraid to use the power of the *spoken* word to intersect and overcome persistent internal negative self-talk. If you are having a hard time internally replacing a negative thought with a positive one, take a deep breath, and speak out loud with conviction, energy, and enthusiasm. Hearing yourself speak positively can have a powerful internal effect and help you achieve proper internal self-talk. Don't be afraid to literally shout out in the middle of a workout, "Yes, I can do it!"

PRACTICING THE POWER OF SELF-TALK

The basics of self-talk and sports psychology are being used right now with elite law-enforcement agencies and Special Forces as well as professional sports teams. To increase performance within the extreme nature of their operations, they are taught techniques in goal-setting, microgoals, "arousal control" using breathing techniques like box breathing, visualization of successful execution and outcomes, and positive self-talk habits.

Your daily Firebreather workouts are ideal opportunities to develop and sharpen this mental skill and create a habit of positive self-talk. Two simple self-talk practices, affirmations and first words, will help you implement this all-powerful skill in the course of your daily life.

TEN AFFIRMATIONS FOR A POSITIVE MIND-SET

Before and during a workout, keep on the alert for negative thoughts slipping into the loop. If you catch one, identify it and replace it. Even better, work on avoiding them altogether by repeating one of these positive mantras over and over, building up a firewall against intrusion.

1. I believe in myself, and I love myself, and I constantly reaffirm my ability to succeed. (I created this affirmation for UFC legend Gray Maynard and Brazilian Jiu-Jitsu Black Belt World Champion Nathan Mendelsohn.)
2. I am protected and surrounded by spiritual light and energy that resonates with courage, confidence, self-esteem, and self-love.
3. I am loved and supported by God (Spirit, Universe, etc.) in the pursuit of my divine life purpose.
4. My mind, body, and spirit are in a state of perfect integration and expression.
5. I resonate and calibrate with universal intelligence, radiant health, and a perfect state of well-being.
6. My mind-set is alive with positive expectancy, encouraging self-talk and optimism.
7. I can overcome any challenge set before me.
8. I believe unconditionally in myself and in the ability of others.
9. I am in alignment with perfect technique, range of motion, and performance principles.
10. I love the challenge.

FIRST WORDS

The first words we speak each day are not to be wasted. They have vital and profound impact. When you wake up, your mind is like the flat surface of a pond. You want to toss the right stone into the center of that pond, so that the ripples that flow from it help you set the right energy and direction for the day.

Upon awakening, I embrace the stillness and silence of the moment. Without speaking, I move quietly to the kitchen and pour a glass of water.

As I drink, I allow a feeling of gratitude for the water. I then shift to an awareness of my breathing and might perform alternate nostril breathing. I then move to a place to sit and conduct a simple and brief seated medita-

EARLY LESSONS IN SELF-TALK

When I was growing up, my dad constantly reinforced the power of the spoken word to my brothers and me. He encouraged us to use words in a constructive way, and to only bring into the universe ideas that were consistent with love, opportunity, and positive action.

My dad knew that I wanted to serve in law-enforcement and military professions. Concerned that I would only embrace the physical aspects of these careers, my dad offered me some sound wisdom: "Greg, a true warrior does more than wear a uniform and carry a weapon. A true warrior speaks a language of infinite possibility and positive expectancy. A true warrior guards their words, and has the courage to correct the language of others."

My father was a chiropractor, pastor, lifeguard, swim coach, body-builder, Naval officer, and athletic trainer. To date, he was the most physically fit man I have ever known. He inspired in me at a very young age the significance of having a strong and robust physical body. He believed that human beings were made to serve one another and viewed the physical body as a tool that could be used for the benefit of the world. By developing a strong and capable body, we were better able to help other people in times of need.

He spoke often about the power of thoughts, and how positive thoughts manifested themselves in positive physical actions. By turn, positive actions created positive thought and emotions.

My father always had a smile on his face. His posture was always supremely straight and he walked with a bounce in his step. The physical body and actions he displayed were complemented by his words and indeed by his very thoughts. He spoke positively about the world, all those he had contact with, and about himself.

tion, my mind aware of the inward and outward flow of breath.

From this stillness, I allow the words to form in my mind that will be my first spoken words of the day. These words are chosen carefully, breaking the morning silence in a self-affirming way.

When I teach yoga, I refer to this practice as "the warrior practice of first words." I cue students in my class as they come out of the final resting pose to practice first words, saying the following: "I encourage you now to practice the warrior tradition of first words. The practice is such that when you speak, you imagine your spoken word rippling through the fertile soil of the universe, ultimately manifesting and touching every corner of your life. Therefore, speak your first words with light, love, and positive expectancy."

Keep in mind that every time you speak, you are speaking into silence. Therefore, first words are most powerful in the morning, because of the length of time you have been in silence. However, even in the middle of a heated conversation, you can take a breath, internally pause, and then practice first words.

Personally, I always break the sacred silence of the early morning hours with a Bible verse. However, your first words can be inspired from within the wisdom of your soul. Just ensure, as I teach in yoga, that your first words are always offered with "light, love, and positive expectancy."

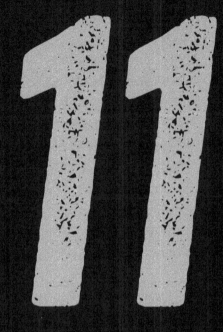

RECHANNELING YOUR THOUGHTS

ANOTHER CRITICAL MENTAL TOOL is specifically aimed at managing fear. Microgoals and self-talk are also powerful in this regard, especially when you're actively in the middle of a tough endeavor. But rechanneling your thoughts involves arming yourself *beforehand*—before a workout, a contest, or any endeavor that provokes fear or worry. To head fear off at the pass, before it can take hold, you must learn to recognize and let go of what you don't have control over and channel that energy into what you do have control over.

Giving a speech, for example, can be scary for many people. The idea of standing up in front of a large group and talking can enable all sorts of worry and fears in the hours or days prior. Images of making mistakes or coming off poorly will feed the dog of fear like you're forking over T-bone steaks. The result can be paralyzing—you may not be able to focus on anything else in the hours leading up to the speech.

In the first years of CrossFit seminars, many people who attended had their doubts about the program. One of my jobs at a seminar was to compete, head-to-head, against the skeptics. I never knew when it was coming but it would come: I would be called upon to perform the infamous workout known as Fran against a visitor.

Fran is a CrossFit workout that is perhaps the most feared and anxiety-provoking benchmark workout there is. It's three rounds of pull-ups and thrusters, performed at the best speed you can summon. At rounds of 21 reps, 15 reps, and 9 reps of each exercise, it doesn't look too bad on paper. But in execution at a fast, hard pace—well, let me put it this way: If there's one workout that is a good bet to make you feel like throwing up, this is probably it.

I felt a great deal of fear and pressure about this task. I would have trouble sleeping the night before a seminar because I had no idea when it was going to happen. It might happen in the first hour of the seminar, or the last. Or somewhere in between. Also, I had no idea if the person I would be competing against would be an amazing Firebreather himself, who would put me to the test and maybe beat me. Finally, I was intensely loyal to Greg Glassman, and I didn't want to let him down. My job was to defend the program and I felt pressure from that.

So in the hours before the moment that I would be called upon to perform Fran, my energy was often drained away by anxiety over questions that couldn't be answered: When was it going to happen? Who would I be competing against? Would I be good enough so that I don't embarrass my coach and the program?

I went through this ordeal hundreds of times. But I was fortunate, because along with my education in CrossFit I was also practicing various martial arts with tremendous teachers. To deal with my fear and worry, I began to apply what I had learned in arts such as jiu-jitsu, karate, and Aikido about energy, or "chi."

Using methods such as deep breathing, positive self-talk, consciously remaining in the present, and focusing on good communication with stu-

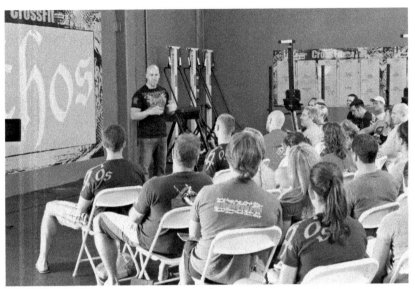

The first official CrossFit Goal Setting Seminar was in 2010 at CrossFit Ethos in Rancho Cucamonga.

dents at the seminar, I was able to let go and re-channel my chi. In addition, I proactively armed myself against fear by ensuring that I was training hard in the week prior to be as prepared as possible, and making choices to eat well, sleep well, and perform my warm-up.

Learning to set my focus on what I could control in place of what I could not had a tremendous impact on not only my experience in CrossFit seminars but also my performance in law enforcement. In the early part of my career, my mind was often swept into things I had no control over. Being in a state of fear has consequences when you're engaged with a parolee or potentially violent suspects. Especially those charged up on drugs. They can be utterly fearless, capable of anything. My fear or doubt could be picked up upon and would encourage their impulse to attack.

As I began to separate the items I should dwell upon from items beyond my control, and shifted thoughts and awareness to those things under my influence, I became more rooted in the present. Energy was conserved rather than fretted away. And my work performance improved.

Learn to recognize and let go of what you don't have control over and channel that energy into what you have influence over.

You can begin using this tool today.

First, cultivate awareness. In other words, pay attention to what you're paying attention to. Especially when you feel your "fight or flight" anxiety heating up, trace the fear to the thoughts behind it. Are you obsessing about what may or may not happen in the future? Worrying over items beyond your control?

Next, gently acknowledge the direction of your fearful thoughts and shift them to an area within your control. If it's a speech, take that energy and use it to do another practice run. Before a hard workout, shift that energy to something you can control: for example, a solid warm-up.

Especially at the beginning, it can be helpful to envision this process in a tangible way. Try drawing two large circles, on a poster board or in a journal, to help distinguish between those things you can control and those you can't. Then choose to keep your mind—along with positive self-talk techniques and microgoals—centered on those things that are yours to control.

BRINGING MIND INTO ALIGNMENT

In 2004, Coach Glassman, Josh Everett, and I traveled to Fort Lewis, Washington, to teach a CrossFit seminar to the 19th Special Forces Group. It was a brutal three days of training. It was December, and all the workouts were outdoors at elevation. By Sunday I was completely exhausted, and so were the tough-as-nails soldiers we were training. Finally, the last workout of the seminar was upon us. After Coach Glassman briefed the workout, he looked at Captain Perry, the senior officer of the group, and said, "Sir, I want you to pick five of your men to complete this final workout. If these five finish under the time cap, then nobody else will have to do the workout. If they fail, everyone has to do the workout."

I was terrified, silently hoping that Captain Perry would not pick me. I wondered how he could pick anyone. Indeed, all the soldiers, along with Josh and myself, could barely stand up. Hunched over, with hands on our knees and labored breathing, everyone's gaze was on the ground. I looked at Captain Perry, interested to see what he would do in this moment.

Just then, an amazing act of leadership and mental toughness unfolded before me. Captain Perry looked around at the group. Then he stood up, rolled his shoulders back, and took a deep breath. Standing tall, with head held high, Perry said in a commanding voice, "It's OK, men. I've got this one. I will do the final workout." With that, Captain Perry bent over, hoisted two huge sandbags, and took off into the final workout.

What do you think the other soldiers did? Every one of us stood up, took a deep breath, and then hoisted our own sandbags, taking off in a full sprint after Captain Perry. We all finished well under the time limit.

Following the workout, I went up to Captain Perry and said, "Sir, that was incredible. You just transformed a group of guys who were defeated. Tell me what you did, and how you did it."

To this, Captain Perry said a few words I will always remember: "Greg, when I looked around at the group, I realized we were all in a position of defeat. I knew I needed to place my body into a position of power that my mind would follow."

The simplicity of his advice has stayed with me, and I use and teach it to this day. When breathing is full and deep, and posture is upright, it is much easier to bring our thinking and mind-set into alignment with our goals. With an integrated training program, you begin to see how the mind affects the body, how the body affects the mind, and how when the body and mind are perfectly connected, our spirit is able to shine.

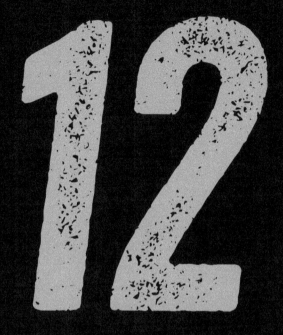

12

BREATHING
THROUGH STRESS

REAL LIFE IS FULL OF STRESSORS. So instead of focusing on being stress-free, which isn't possible and thus doomed to end in frustration, we are better off investigating the nature of the stress, and considering how the stress affects our body, mind, and spirit.

The final instrument in your mental-strength toolbox, one that will assist you in dealing with stress and refocusing thoughts on to those things within your influence, is one you have had along with you since the day you were born: breathing.

A series of deep breaths is extremely powerful. Putting your attention into a good, deep belly breath forces you into the present moment, clearing your mind and taking the edge off your distress.

Again, it was Mark Divine, one of my key mentors, who helped me embrace this lesson. Although breathing had been a part of my martial arts training for years, it was in facing a particular terror I had that showed me how powerful an asset a good, deep breath can be.

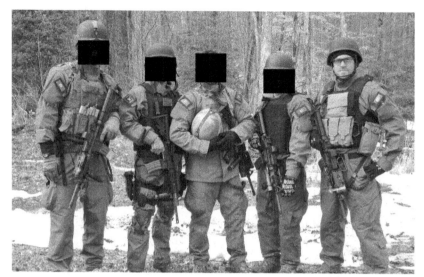

Among brothers and warriors during the Foreign-deployed Advisory and Support Team (FAST) Selection and Assessment Course in Quantico, Virginia. This was one of the most challenging crucibles of my life.

In 2010 I was preparing to attend the DEA Foreign-deployed Advisory and Support Team (FAST) 30-day assessment and selection course in Quantico, Virginia. The course would be 30 days of intense training evolutions designed to test the mental and physical limits of the candidates in attendance. I knew the course would include rappelling, fast roping from a helicopter, and various other evolutions in which height would play a factor.

And I was afraid of heights.

I called Mark and asked if he could help prepare me for the FAST course, specifically the evolutions involving heights. Mark agreed and told me to meet him the following weekend at the Navy SEAL obstacle course in Coronado, California. On an early Saturday morning, I met Mark on the sand at the outskirts of the SEAL compound. I saw, looming ominously in the distance, several obstacles reaching high into the sky. Without much fanfare or conversation, Mark said, "Follow me, Greg" and took off in a dead sprint through the deep sand toward the gate to the obstacle course.

Half a mile later, Mark and I were at the base of the 50-foot cargo net. No directions, no points of performance, no safety brief.

Mark shouted, "Hooyah! Stay next to me Greg," and started climbing.

I continued up the cargo net next to Mark. He took the inside position, and I climbed on the outside, with a large wood telephone-pole-like beam on my right side, the ocean just beyond. At the top of the net, 50 feet off the ground, we stopped. I looked up and noticed a frightening 2-foot gap between the end of the cargo net and another wooden crossbeam. To me, that 2-foot gap seemed larger than life, and I desperately hoped that all we'd do next was climb back down, the same way we had come up. I had a death grip on the rope of the cargo net, and I was staring straight ahead. My breath was shallow and fast, and my mind was racing.

Mark, with impeccable timing, said, "Greg, now would be a good time to take a deep breath."

He was exactly right. I needed to breathe deeply and take back control of my mind. I forced a deep breath in through my nose, and a slow breath out through my mouth. My field of vision opened a bit, and I felt my body—and my grip—begin to relax slightly.

"The next step is to climb up and over that wood beam, and then down the other side of the net."

My breathing raced again, and I locked down on the rope.

"Greg, I want you to point to what is causing you stress," Mark said.

His question snapped me into the present moment. I realized the stress was actually *not* the height I was off the ground; it was *not* the 2-foot gap between the net and the wood beam; it was *not* the task of climbing over the beam; it was *not* even the fear of falling to the ground, 50 feet below. An honest assessment of that moment resulted in the sudden realization that the cause of the stress was not, in fact, any external factor at all.

When you change your thinking about what you are perceiving, what you are perceiving begins to change.

It existed in one place: inside my mind.

The stress I was experiencing was taking place solely in my mind, and it centered on my thoughts about the height, falling, and traversing the wood beam. Ah! This was an empowering revelation. For if I could change my thoughts, I could change my feelings and my actions.

With another deep, even, and calm breath, Mark and I smiled at one another, appreciating the moment of awareness I had achieved. I climbed up and over the wood beam, came face to face with Mark, shouted "Hooyah!" and then climbed down the other side.

During the FAST assessment and selection course, I used this lesson during the fast-roping and rappelling evolutions. Specifically, during a final testing evaluation involving a 50-foot fast rope from a helicopter onto a shoot-house rooftop, I took a deep breath and reminded myself that any stress I was experiencing was only in my mind. If I could create stress in the form of fear, I could also cultivate courage, determination, and focus. With a deep breath, I gripped the fast rope, swung out the door, and slid safely down the rope, joining my team on the rooftop below.

I learned a two-step process that morning in Coronado, and I share it with you here. It is a powerful tool to use when combating anxiety and acute fears while en route to difficult, important goals.

Breathe deeply: We can't breathe in the past, and we can't breathe in the future. We breathe in the present moment. Deep breathing brings you into the present moment and helps create space between the stimulus you are experiencing and your reaction to it.

Point to the cause of the stress: Remind yourself that the cause of the stress is not external to your experience. Rather, turn attention inward to the quality of your thinking, and know that it is shaping your perspective of what you are experiencing. When you change your thinking about what you are perceiving, what you are perceiving begins to change.

Deep breathing brings you into the present moment and helps create space between the stimulus you are experiencing and your reaction to it.

Martial arts, yoga, and meditation all begin with the centering power and energy flow of the breath. Why? Because breathing is both grounding and energizing.

Breathing is also a point where the mental, physical, and spiritual come together. And there, your Firebreathing truly begins.

SPIRIT

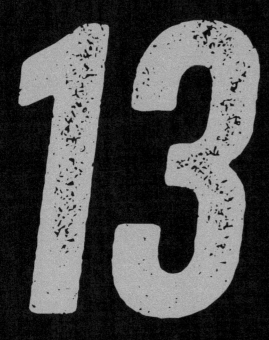

13

BUILDING A
SPIRITUAL PRACTICE

DR. KELLY STARRETT IS A BEST-SELLING AUTHOR and the creator of the MobilityWOD website, where he offers up an encyclopedia's worth of education and problem-solving on how to improve positions, movement, and power output. Kelly has a global following and consults with NFL teams, top MLB players, Tour de France cyclists, and Special Operations teams from both military and law enforcement.

During speaking engagements, Kelly often poses a question to the audience: *Do you have a movement practice?* For him, having a movement practice such as yoga or Pilates means dedicating a block of time to working toward improving your mobility and your ability to assume and hold good positions. You might have your sport—cycling, rowing, basketball, surfing—and that's great. But to support your sport and your life in general, Kelly advises people to build a movement practice.

Kelly's question—the motivation behind it and the importance he places upon it—makes a helpful entryway into our discussion of the spiritual dimension of Firebreather Fitness. For, just as Kelly suggests that you should find a movement practice that supports you and your sport, I am advocating that you find a spiritual practice that does the same. So my first question for you is this: *Do you have a spiritual practice?*

I am not here to advocate a particular religious or spiritual practice. I'm a Christian, and so that is an important part of my personal spiritual practice. That is what's right for me. However, as renowned yoga teacher Rolf Gates once told me, "All spiritual paths ultimately lead to the light." Christianity has been the right path for me, but it might not be right for you. What I am asking you to find is the spiritual path that speaks to your heart and moral compass, and then you can dedicate yourself to that pursuit.

While it may seem odd to emphasize the value and importance of mind/body/spirit as opposed to simply mind/body, I would argue that it's not only a natural fit, it is an optimal one. There is no achieving optimal physical performance without a spiritual practice. Just no way. Furthermore, in order to express your unique purpose and achieve peak performance both in the gym and, more importantly, in life, a dedicated spiritual practice is vital.

So let's cut to a simple, practical example within the context of exercise. When physical training gets extremely hard and uncomfortable, how do you keep going? When you're in the middle of an especially tough workout and a negative voice in your head suggests it's time to quit, where do you dig? During any challenging circumstance, whether in life or sport, when everything seems stacked against you, how do you maintain personal belief and keep marching forward? Outside the gym, how do you respond to the challenges that life presents to you? When there's loss and hardship, even tragedy, and those supreme difficulties that are a part of being human become your testing ground, how do you maintain your life path, intentions, and goals? Oftentimes in life, the strength we need to cultivate and rely on most lies in the spiritual realm.

And what about the long haul? What energizes that purpose we discussed in Chapter 8, such that you can sustain your chosen disciplines for

Oftentimes in life, the strength we need to cultivate and rely on most lies in the spiritual realm.

weeks, months, years? Or charges you up for the sequence of challenges you choose to take on, such as the Firebreather Fitness plan? Anyone can get through one workout. But what about ten? Or 100? Or 1,000? What is it that you truly want to achieve from those pursuits? It is probably more than just six-pack abs and bragging rights. The truly valuable challenges that we choose to embrace in life exist much deeper within us. They feed and are fed by our spirit. Many of the challenges we seek out, on the playing field, in the gym, and in life, are about fully realizing who we are and what we're capable of.

The sport of ultramarathon—running events that are upwards of 100 miles long—continues to gain popularity. Why the draw? Why run for 24 hours straight (or more!)? The reason doesn't begin and end with being physically fit. After all, ultramarathons are not the kind of athletic endeavor that directly improves your physical health. In fact, they are actually hard on the muscles, skeleton, and body chemistry.

So why do it? As many runners will tell you, the draw of running an ultramarathon has roots in the spiritual domain. At some point in the race, after a great deal of physical and mental exhaustion, things get stripped down to a point where it becomes almost completely a spiritual exercise. This was the same experience many of the Kokoro candidates and I encountered during the mental and physical ordeals imposed on us during nearly 50 continual hours of physical training evolutions. At a certain point, the senses and mind turn inward, drawing on a strength, resolve, and inner purpose that ultimately provides the foundation we need most.

Other sports have a spiritual draw, especially those that connect you with nature, such as surfing, kayaking, mountain biking, and climbing.

I have experience in a number of these sports, as well as a 20-year practice of martial arts and a deep study of yoga. I have also led a professional life dedicated to the protection and service of others. All of these, which have a place in the spiritual realm, have sharpened my approach to being a Fire-breather, making me not just a better athlete, but a more fulfilled human.

There are different approaches in teaching the martial arts. I've had training in a variety, including Brazilian jiu-jitsu, karate, Krav Maga, and Aikido. I first learned Aikido with my dad. My dad was opposed to violence, and so, not surprisingly, he was drawn to the core lesson in Aikido, which reflects this: Don't resist force with force.

And yet Aikido was highly valuable training for my work in the law-enforcement profession. Indeed, this teaching would eventually be at the heart of my approach to police work. Understanding the principles of Aikido helped me simultaneously increase my effectiveness as a peace officer while minimizing the use and risk of violent measures, like pepper spray, a baton, or a gun.

As part of my own spiritual practice, and having embodied the teachings that my dad encouraged, with values like forgiveness and goodwill, I worked to find a solution to the conflict between taking a nonviolent stance and being in law enforcement, where violent confrontations are inevitable.

It didn't come easily. In my first years of service, this conflict inhibited my performance. I was apprehensive and fearful, especially when pursuing parolees or suspects that were physically stronger or hopped up on drugs. This fear inhibited me when confronting those who feared no one; who believed they had little to lose, and would rather risk their life than return to prison. The fear I was experiencing had less to do with physical injury to myself, and more a fear of violating a value that had been instilled in me by my faith: Love your neighbor as you love yourself.

During my early CrossFit training, around 2003, Greg Glassman talked about how martial arts training might be the program's tip of the spear. It was at that time, too, that my study of karate introduced me to samurais and their unique warrior culture. Two books were powerfully influential for me: *The Art of War* by Sun Tzu and *The Book of Five Rings* by Miyamoto Musashi.

Although their titles give the impression these books are all about fighting and inflicting maximum violence with a weapon, they are more about tactics and how to win a fight without ever drawing a weapon. There was a heavy emphasis on the spiritual dimension. I later began to understand that the spirituality in disciplines like yoga and certain martial arts were within this same vein.

In *The Book of Five Rings*, Musashi writes: "In strategy your spiritual bearing must not be any different from normal. Both in fighting and in everyday life you should be determined though calm."

Calmness, stillness, tranquility, and spiritual equilibrium—Musashi's philosophy encourages building a physical and mental skill set on a spiritual foundation.

Both books have readerships that go well beyond a military crowd. For business leaders, coaches, and athletes seeking to become the best at what they do, the principles are of tremendous value.

My personal and professional experimentation with applying these ideas showed me that they work as well now as they did centuries ago. In my role as a peace officer, the more I understood and practiced these principles—calmness, stillness, tranquility, spiritual equilibrium—in my daily beat on patrol, the more I was able to bring peaceful conclusions to what otherwise might have been violent interactions. By intentionally and habitually including a spiritual practice into my daily life, and combining my physical, mental, and spiritual training, I found that I was no longer held back by fear. I wasn't draining my willpower and capacities by being off-balance and uncertain.

In this new, integrated state of body-mind-spirit presence, I operated tactically. Rather than wait for smoldering situations to burst into violence, I proactively met with gang leaders and had one-to-one, honest, direct conversations. The power of this approach was remarkable. My being honest and direct triggered their honest and direct responses. It often had the power to disarm my foes, literally and figuratively. Using this new tactic, battles were often won before even a single provocative word

HOLD YOUR HEAD UP!

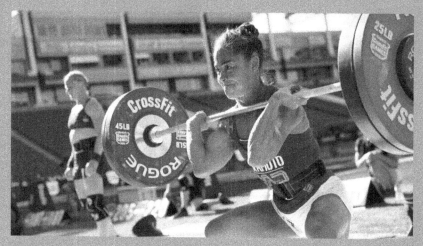

There is a simple technique that my friend, elite CrossFit star athlete and coach, Annie Sakamoto, puts to use both in the rigorous workouts she charges into, as well as in competitions. It's a principle of movement and position that Kelly Starrett talks about as well, and it suggests the nature of how body, mind, and spirit are all part of the whole.

Annie's resolve and competitive ferocity are legendary. She goes at her workouts with the energy and spirit of an Olympic gymnast. When she's busy tearing through one of her signature over-the-red-line efforts and a wave of metabolic fatigue slams into her, she resists the temptation to bend, drop her hands down onto her knees, or take any other physical position that signals "I'm beat." Rather, if forced to take a rest, she will do so in a very controlled manner, and always while retaining a strong physical posture. This simple discipline has a powerful effect on her resolve, energy, and force. She has tuned into the fact that her choice of physical position for recovery is powerful. Slump over and the spirit slumps with you. Stand tall and strong and the spirit stands tall and strong with you.

Musashi talks about this tactic in The Book of Five Rings: "Adopt a stance with the head erect, neither hanging down, nor looking up, nor twisted." Adopt this simple technique in your Firebreather training workouts. Pay attention to the flow of energy, calmness, and power when you sustain positions and postures suggesting power and energy.

was uttered, let alone a fist clenched or weapon drawn. When I absolutely had to use force to protect myself or apprehend an aggressive offender, I did so without malice or an intention for violence. Instead, with a sense of love and commitment to the duty of my sworn oath, I relied on technique, leverage, and strategy to overcome the most intense resistance without injury to myself or others. My integration of my mind, body, and spirit had positive, winning results in my profession.

Making a spiritual practice a priority in your fitness program is like creating an energy field around you.

You may or may not face this particular kind of danger in your own life, but let me assure you that whatever your battles and challenges, making a spiritual practice a priority in your fitness program is like creating an energy field around you. A spiritual practice helps tie it all together— that hard workout, your purpose, the daily drumbeat of your self-talk— unifying these practices into a singular and powerful program for fitness and for life.

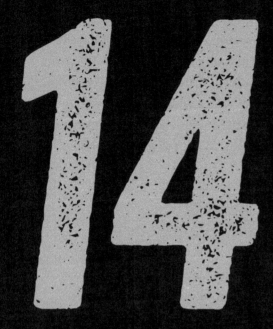

14

BUILDING STRENGTH AND RESILIENCE

SETTING BIG GOALS, executing tough workouts, moving actively toward your purpose: These all require large doses of strength and resiliency. Integrating a spiritual practice into your workouts will help you find that inner strength when the physical road throws up barriers and stressors.

In this chapter we will talk about a few simple, direct methods you can add to your program so that your Firebreather workouts reap the benefits of a spiritual discipline.

The most simple yet effective techniques to hone strength and resiliency are those aimed at **stress reduction**. Combating stress in order to relax the body and quiet the mind builds your spiritual strength and aids your workouts.

The majority of the great spiritual texts and disciplines teach that the fundamental cause of suffering is the mind's tendency to either regress to the past or project itself into the future. The solution, therefore, is to discipline the mind to remain centered in the present moment. During meditation, this tendency of the mind to leap out of the present moment becomes extremely apparent. Indeed, holding the attention on the present moment can seem harder than the most demanding physical workout. In many respects, learning to "work in" is more challenging, and more important, than learning to "work out."

The solution is to discipline the mind to remain centered in the present moment.

In my military and law-enforcement career, I noticed how easy it was for my mind to project itself into the future and to worry about what might happen. In these moments, because my mind was resting on a future creation that had no bearing in the present moment, I was unaware of my body and my breath. As a result, my body was tight and my breathing was shallow, which only exaggerated the mental sensations I was entertaining. Learning to remain present, with the mind continually realigning to the body and the breath, is a powerful practice that can have a profoundly positive effect on your workouts, career, and life.

Remaining present helps you gain perspective on what is permanent versus what is temporary. When we become still and silent, and begin to witness our thoughts, we awaken the part of our consciousness I refer to as the "great witness." This ability to create a little bit of space between our thoughts and our great witness helps us to discern where we are focusing our attention. Your mind is like a giant magnifying glass, and what you focus on will therefore tend to increase in your life. When you focus on a problem, the problem only increases. The real insight here, however, is that the majority of the time, the problem we are focusing on is our *perception* of a situation, and not the situation itself. It's our thinking that determines the quality of what we are seeing. And when we change the way we look at something, what we look at begins to change. Everything begins in the temple of our mind.

A strong spiritual practice helps cultivate your ability to meet and greet stress in the present, as it arises in your consciousness. Engaging stress as a Firebreather means dealing with it on the field of battle at the moment the stress presents itself. In this context, that stress can actually turn into a strengthening experience and an opportunity to discipline yourself to remain in the present moment.

Breathing is another valuable tool that will keep you in the present. The practice of watching the breath teaches stability and helps the mind discover what action can be taken in the present, and what illusions of the future, or memories of the past, need to be resolved.

In yoga, we bring awareness to the four parts of the breath: the inhalation, retention of the breath after inhalation, exhalation, and suspension of the breath after exhalation. The in-breath should be long, slow, subtle, deep, and evenly spread throughout the body. The in-breath draws energy from the atmosphere into the cells of the lungs, and rejuvenates and restores the life force within us. By retaining the breath once drawn in, the energy is fully absorbed and evenly distributed through all the systems of the body through the circulation of blood. The slow release of air during exhalation carries out accumulated toxins, both mental and physical. By pausing after the out-breath to a level of comfort unique to the moment, all mental stresses are purged away, and the mind is naturally drawn to the present moment.

As you continue to draw your attention to the inner movement of the breath, and become sensitive to each of the four parts of the breath, it becomes impossible for your awareness to remain attached to the external senses, the past, or the future. Even one brief moment of absolutely present moment awareness is enough to release the grasp of the past, or the tempting pull of the future. Meditation on the breath is a powerful step in the withdrawal from the external engagement of the mind with the memories of the past or the tendency to plan, wrestle with, or be concerned for the future.

Let's use an example from the gym to see how withdrawing from the external engagement of the mind can help you achieve satisfaction and benefit from physical training. In the early days of my CrossFit training, I would experience a lot of stress and anxiety as Coach Glassman approached the whiteboard and began to write out the workout of the day (WOD). Because I did not know what he was going to prescribe, my mind raced with "what if" scenarios. My body and breathing were trying to keep up with my mind, and as a result, my body was tense and my breath was rapid. Although I was stressing over the unknown nature of the workout I would soon face, I noticed that my training partner Loyd Lewis always seemed tranquil and unaffected. Eager to learn his secret, I asked him one morning, "Loyd, brother, how do you remain so calm when I am so stressed over the upcoming workout?" Loyd's response provided me with one of the greatest insights I've ever received: "It's easy, man. I simply keep my mind focused on what I can influence." In that moment, I realized why it was key to remain focused on the present moment, both in the gym and in life. When our minds leap into the future, or retreat into the past, we get stuck, because our bodies are *here* and *now*, while our mind is somewhere else. And because we are here and now, we can only affect the present moment. And what's always in the present moment? Our body and our breath. This is why maintaining awareness of our breathing and our posture is so important. Our body and breath are like an anchor for our spirit, helping to keep us securely grounded in the present moment.

Being present with a clear and quiet mind has proven benefits on performance. Former Navy SEAL Kirk Parsley, MD, who works with active-duty SEALs on health and performance, gives a talk about how performance and willpower are drained if you allow your thoughts to be swept off by insignificant thinking and wasteful decision-making. Parsley says that after a good night's sleep, we wake up in the morning fully recharged with willpower. But if the first thing you do is to pick up your smartphone and start scrolling through your e-mail, you're already starting to drain your willpower battery in a wasteful way. Even seemingly insignificant distractions and decisions exhaust this critical source. Learning about the science that Dr. Parsley lectures about makes sense to me: I'm sure, for example, that one of the reasons I've been successful with nutrition is that I structured it so that as many decisions as possible were already made and turned into routines and habits. Developing intentional rituals and processes so that you stay present and using breathing and meditation to ward off unnecessary stress and keep your mind quiet will pay off huge dividends when it comes to spending that daily dose of willpower on the things you really want to spend it on. Like a Firebreather Fitness workout.

BREATHING

In the following chapter, we will explore more deeply the practice and benefits of yoga, but let's start here with a few yogic-style breathing techniques, which are in themselves meditations. Use these techniques to clear stress from your mind and body and replace it with a spiritual type of energy.

You can use these in moments of daily frustration, such as being stuck in a long line at the grocery store or in bad traffic on the freeway. In addition, these techniques work wonders in the midst of a challenging workout, or when confronted with a challenging life circumstance.

I am a big believer that the gym, yoga studio, or martial arts dojo is a training ground where we can cultivate the skills that we need to be at our best in life. Your physical Firebreather training sessions are outstanding opportunities to consistently practice breathing exercises before the start of a workout in order to get your mind into the present, prepared and focused to give maximum effort. These are also useful when negative thoughts creep in during a hard workout, as they inevitably do. Effective breathing techniques can metaphorically "blow negativity out of your mind." Then you can fill that space with positive self-talk power statements. You'll be gaining multiple benefits: You'll increase the effectiveness of your workouts and also build and reinforce the habits you want when other stressful moments happen during an average day.

Here are my favorite breathing exercises. Mastering them takes a little practice, but you will find soon enough that they begin to feel quite natural.

BOX BREATHING

When I was assigned to my first duty station in El Centro, California, as a brand new DEA special agent, I had the opportunity to attend a lecture by renowned author and educator Colonel David Grossman. David is a retired Army Ranger who is deeply respected in the warrior professions for his commitment to teaching the power of the mind and the benefits of a specific breathing practice. During the lecture, David explained the breathing practice he calls "combat breathing," which is a four-count breathing exercise that helps calm the mind and trigger the body's parasympathetic nervous system. This system, referred to as "rest and digest," is an important contrast to the predominant sympathetic nervous system that most law enforcement and military operators tend to exist in. The sympathetic nervous system, often referred to as "flight or fight," is preparing the body for survival. This system is absolutely necessary during moments when we have to physically protect ourselves or others from a threat to our personal safety. However, due to the power of the mind, we can unintentionally remain fixed in this state if we are worrying about the future or trying to change something that's happened in the past. The combat breathing technique centers the mind in the present moment and results in increased states of relaxation, mental calm, and focus.

Although I enjoyed the lecture, I did not continue to practice the technique and soon forgot the important lesson Colonel Grossman had provided. Thankfully, I had another opportunity to learn and practice this technique during Kokoro Camp in 2010. Sometime during the first 10 hours of the brutal, nonstop calisthenics and cold-water immersion tests, retired

Navy SEAL commander Mark Divine, author of *The Way of the SEAL: Think Like an Elite Warrior to Lead and Succeed*, taught my boat crew the fundamentals of breathing, which were the same technique taught by Colonel Grossman. Mark refers to it as "box breathing," which I like because the image of my breathing making a box was very helpful. I committed myself to the daily practice of box breathing and discovered within just a few weeks of using the technique an increased sense of inner peace and an ability to remain present, even during the stress of a tough physical workout or a dangerous mission with the DEA.

Box breathing is simple to learn and to begin using right now. The technique is as follows:

*Breathe in through the nose for four counts . . .
hold for four counts . . . breathe out through the nose for four counts
. . . hold for four counts. Complete four rounds.*

The nostril breathing, combined with combat breathing or box breathing, has several additional benefits. The hair follicles in the nose help to either warm or cool the air, and clean the air before entering your lungs. The nostril breath also tends to "pull the breath" into the lower diaphragm, filling the lungs from the bottom to the top. Finally, the nostril breath triggers the parasympathetic nervous system.

Notice how you feel, both mentally and physically, after four rounds of box breathing. Note the dual feelings of stress melting away and energy being drawn into the lungs and through the body. As you gently center your mind on the movement of your breath, notice how you are realigning with the present moment.

Over the next few days, whenever you feel your temperature rising from accumulated stress or unintentional negative self-talk, shift into box breathing mode. Watch frustration and anxiety burn away while positive energy, faith, and optimism flow in.

ADVANCED BREATHING TECHNIQUES

Another series of breathing techniques are more advanced. Think of box breathing as your physical squat. It is an essential skill that will increase your power in the mental and spiritual realm. The techniques that follow are more like your handstand push-ups and overhead squat. They are more advanced, yet when practiced and developed will yield huge benefits. These breathing techniques come from Ashtanga yoga, and are written in Sankskrit.

Nadi shodhana (alternate nostril breathing)

Gently exhale all the air from your lungs. Close the right nostril with the thumb of the right hand, and inhale slowly and deeply through left nostril. Close the left nostril with the right ring finger, releasing the thumb, and exhale through the right. Inhale through the right, then close it with the thumb and exhale through the left. This makes one round. Complete 10 rounds.

Dirgha Rechak (long exhaled breath)

Inhale normally, then exhale as slowly and smoothly as possible. Concentrate on the exhale, making it long, smooth, and subtle. Inhale again normally, and start another round. Complete 10 rounds.

Dirgha Purak (long inhaled breath)

Exhale normally, then inhale as slowly and smoothly as possible. Concentrate on the inhale, making it long, smooth, and subtle. Exhale normally, and start another round. Complete 10 rounds.

BASIC MEDITATION

In yoga and in the martial arts, meditation is a discipline used to quiet the mind and increase awareness of the spiritual realm, both in yourself and in natural surroundings. There are other, hard-science benefits as well: Increasingly, meditation is being used to increase cognitive performance and reduce the ravaging effects of stress. The news of meditation as a method to improve focus and cognitive performance has a generation of adopters across a wide swath, from elite military forces to Silicon Valley CEOs. As you'll see in the Firebreathing 21-day plan, meditation is part of the drumbeat of your daily workout. Meditation within the context of the Firebreather Fitness plan provides the "yoking" or "integrating" element that ultimately links the mind, body, and spirit practices together. During meditation, you are able to unite your values and actions, and calm the turbulence of your mind. Even just a few minutes each day of silence and stillness can have a resounding effect on the quality of not only your workouts but also on your life.

One immediate benefit that a regular meditation practice will have on your training program is mental toughness. Tapping into the bottomless well of inner strength during your daily workouts will enable greater performance, more power, and endurance.

Let's say you're deep into a high-intensity workout designed to last 7 minutes. You're at the halfway point, rotating into a fresh round that starts with 25 kettlebell swings. You're feeling spent. Your breathing and heart rate are skyrocketing. A voice from the pessimistic pit in your mind is trying to get traction. It's trying to lure you into quitting. This is where meditation training can kick in, helping you to let go of negative thoughts, to witness them as things rather than actual forces. This distinction is how you can prevent fear and stress from compounding and taking you down. In elite police and military units, this is called "arousal control." You're in a battle, and this is a moment when your ability to stay calm and steady in the fury of a situation that is both physically and psychologically demanding is critical to performance. The same mechanics apply to your daily workout. When you start to push into the red line, your ability to stay present and work through it without being overcome by fear and stress will help you maximize your results.

One of the best ways to experience the benefits of meditation is to become aware of our energy and to witness the quality of each breath. We tend to think of energy production in the external sense of the word. However, when you become still and silent during meditation, an entirely new world opens to you. You become more aware and sensitive to how closely thoughts and emotions are linked. During the course of our day, we tend to focus on the external objects passing through our field of vision. This draws our energy out into the world. And unfortunately, when focused on the outside world, the mind tends to resist change, working instead to control our external circumstances, forgetting that the external world is in a constant state of change that is outside our ability to control. Meditation helps to reverse this tendency of the mind to attach to the external world, and to reverse the flow of our life force from the outside to the inside. Through steady practice, meditation results in a profound state of peace, for we realize the vast universe within us is the source of everything we had been seeking in the external world.

During an advanced meditation course, master yoga teacher Rolf Gates offered me this visual representation of the effects of meditation: "When you sit down, close your eyes, and become still, the sand begins to settle and the water will become clear." In other words, non-action and non-activity allow us to settle down, and in this settled state, our minds become clear.

But it is important to note that meditation is not necessarily the absence of thoughts. Meditation is, plainly put, the returning of your attention to the meditation. For example, you may choose to focus on your breathing. In this manner, you sit down, close your eyes, and become still. You begin to cultivate your witnessing self, and watch yourself breathe. You essentially witness yourself take a deep breath in, you witness the moment of retained breath, then you witness yourself exhale, and then witness the suspended breath. In the moments that you are absolutely one with your breathing, you are experiencing meditation, and a deep sense of peace will be your natural state.

Sometimes this is easier said than done. The tendency for the mind is the following: You take a deep breath in, then think, "Did I lock my car?"

The mind jumps away from the intended focus of meditation. But rather than judging this experience as negative, your task is to simply take notice and gently return the awareness back to the breath. In doing this you resist the temptation to judge yourself negatively, with negative self-talk or criticism. You just return to the work.

Along with the felt experience of watching my breath, I employ another meditation technique frequently: the repeating of a mantra within my mind. The mantra meditation is wonderful because it allows the mind to enjoy its natural state of activity in a focused manner. For example, the tendency of the mind is to jump from thought to thought, idea to idea, memory to memory. By introducing a mantra, the mind settles around this word, repeating it over and over, until thinking becomes more subtle. In this meditation, it is common to experience internal silence between the thoughts, or what renowned author and meditation advocate Deepak Chopra refers to as "slipping into the gap between your thoughts." The great wisdom teachers instruct that the space between thinking is the universal space of pure awareness—you directly experience the universal mind, pure potentiality, and the unlimited nature of your spirit. In yoga, it is common to use the mantra of the sound "Om," and in my early childhood experience in the Catholic Church, we would repeat the word "Amen."

I recommend meditating at least ten minutes in the morning and ten minutes in the evening. Meditation has been woven into the daily Firebreather Fitness workouts, and in many respects meditation will be the fabric that yokes or joins the mind, body, and spirit practices together. As part of a combined practice, I personally begin each of my meditation sessions with four rounds of box breathing and five rounds of alternate nostril breathing. Although over my life I've practiced daily meditation at varying lengths, I've had the most benefit with two twenty-minute sessions.

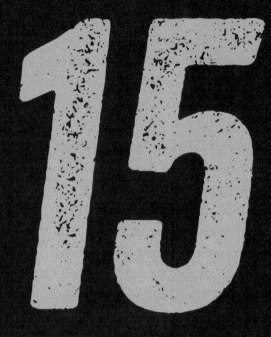

15

YOGA: A PHYSICAL AND SPIRITUAL PRACTICE

I WAS INTRODUCED TO YOGA in a rather peculiar way. It was not at a quiet studio, but rather at Kokoro Camp, invented and conducted by Mark Divine.

Kokoro Camp is a 50-hour experience with no sleep, designed to physically and mentally exhaust the fittest athletes that dare show up. Once fully spent, athletes are forced to begin to dig into their heart and soul in a way that shows that they—all of us—are capable of 20 times what we think we are.

I signed on for the camp in 2010, and after 47 hours of nonstop physical training evolutions, we were instructed to change into dry clothing and gather in the yoga studio at Mark's HQ.

As we sat cross-legged on the studio floor, Mark entered the room and explained the final training evolution: Under constant evaluation by a cadre of combat-proven Navy SEALs, we were instructed to stay awake and focused, and to follow Mark's instruction for two hours of yoga.

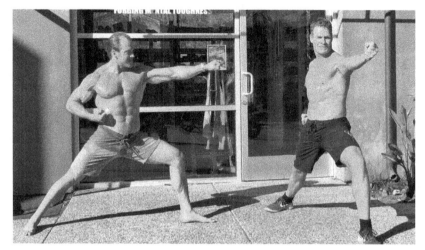

Mark Divine introduced me to yoga during Kokoro Camp. Yoga has been instrumental in my own spiritual practice.

Specifically, we would be led through a warrior yoga practice, which Mark now refers to as Kokoro yoga. Kokoro yoga is Mark's adaptation of the ancient Ashtanga yoga. Its main focus was to develop breath awareness, spinal health, concentration and intuition, and to foster the warrior spirit.

For the next two hours, my classmates and I did our best to follow Mark through a series of traditional yoga poses. With sweat pouring down my entire body, I was astonished at the difficulty of the poses, as well as the stark contrast between the nonstop movement of the previous 47 hours and the stillness and silence of the yoga practice. During the rhythmic flow between postures known as Warrior I and Warrior II, I felt something indescribable release within me, as though a dormant force of immense power had been stirred to life. I knew I wanted to learn more about yoga upon Kokoro graduation.

Finally, after what seemed an eternity of standing poses, balancing poses, inversions, and twisting postures, Mark instructed us to lay down on our backs, in Shavasana, a resting pose also known as corpse pose or dead man's pose. It was an especially sweet feeling, because I, like the other candidates, assumed we had finished Kokoro.

Although the SEAL instructors had warned us to stay awake during warrior yoga, Mark assured the group that during Shavasana, candidates could relax, let go, and allow the integration of the previous two hours of yoga practice to peacefully seep in. Mind you, we'd been awake for more than 47 consecutive hours of nonstop action. I closed my eyes, and within a few seconds, I and the 18 other Kokoro attendees fell soundly asleep on the yoga studio floor.

It was a deception. Kokoro Camp #12 was far from over. Instead, the Navy SEAL instructors had gathered outside the yoga studio, like hornets readying to ambush, waiting for the candidates to fall asleep. As soon as the snoring and sleep twitching started, the instructors burst into the studio, dumping buckets of ice-cold water onto us, and screaming—"How dare you fall asleep! Get yourselves onto the grinder right now!"

It was the mother of rude awakenings, followed by two hours of relentless log drills, calisthenics, ice baths, and ocean immersion. Our class finally heard the words we had been longing for: "Kokoro Class #12, you are secure!"

Afterward, I spoke with Mark about my revelatory experience in yoga. Mark said to me, "Greg, a true warrior must be skillful both in action, and nonaction, both in movement and stillness. This is the benefit of yoga—you can practice both simultaneously."

Intrigued and inspired, I started a six-year journey of my own.

THE MANY LAYERS OF YOGA

No one is quite sure how old yoga is. Scholars suggest it began anywhere from 5,000 to 10,000 years ago. One thing we do know is that yoga wasn't invented as a way to get a beach-ready body. Rather, yoga's roots are intertwined with the martial arts. Yoga, which means "union," is perhaps the first body/mind/spirit program ever invented. One practical value yoga had was that it allowed practitioners of meditation the physical capacity to sit for longer periods.

While certainly a deeply spiritual practice, yoga also offers several key physical benefits.

Body awareness: Yoga provides athletes with deep awareness into how the body moves and feels in space and time. Our senses turn inward, and we deepen the body's intuition. The inner stillness we develop spills over into physical fitness endeavors, including improved quality of movement and virtuosity.

Core development: The core in yoga is built at a very deep and integrated level. We learn how to root into the earth and how to ground ourselves during dynamic movement.

Physical balance: Balancing poses in yoga begin in the mind, then extend through the core, into the earth. Balance in yoga goes beyond typical athletic balance and leads to gracefulness in action, impeccable timing, smoothness of motion, and increased spatial awareness.

Mobility: The deep twisting, bending, and extension work we achieve through yoga poses significantly increases our range of motion and mobility for all athletic endeavors.

Spinal health: The lengthening effect of the standing and bending yoga poses increases space between the vertebra of the spine, reducing a host of injury-related symptoms.

Concentration: Yoga deepens our concentration and our ability to coordinate the movement of the body and breath in action. Yoga has been referred to as a "moving concentration practice."

The first three years of my yoga practice mirrored the first three years of my CrossFit experience. I loved the physicality of the practice and felt my body come alive through the poses. My friendship with Mark Divine continued to grow, and he patiently instructed me. I incorporated a 15-minute routine into my daily CrossFit warm-up, and on rest days I practiced a longer, one-hour routine.

As I grew in my practice and sought to better understand the spiritual aspect of yoga, I was fortunate to receive instruction from Rolf Gates. Rolf is a renowned warrior yogi who leads workshops, seminars, and teacher-trainings, and gives lectures around the world. He wrote the book *Meditations from the Mat.* I had an opportunity in 2014 to take a 200-hour yoga teacher-training course from Rolf at his studio in Santa Cruz. Rolf is a former US Army Ranger and Army captain, which drew me to his style of yoga and way of teaching. Given his background, I anticipated a robust physical practice, similar to my experience on the yoga mat with Mark. However, Rolf's greatest contribution to my yoga practice turned out to be a deepening sense of the inward journey I needed to take. Following are a few of the insights that Rolf gave me. Each time I roll out my mat to practice yoga, I focus on these qualities, which beautifully combine mind, body, and spirit: balance, lightness, extension, and presence.

BALANCE

There was a time I thought a true spiritual path would necessitate a rejection of the world and a turning away from the responsibilities, commitments, and obligations associated with living in it. However, Rolf helped me understand the greater challenge for the spiritual devotee was to live in the world, with all of its trials and tribulations, while at the same time maintaining balance and self-control. Thus, the first spiritual aspect of yoga that Rolf taught me was balance.

Through the consistent practice of yoga, one can begin to develop a perfect balance between both sides of the body, as well as balance among the mind, body, and spirit. Balance in the body does not merely mean standing on one leg or on one's head. Balance in the body is developing balance in every aspect of life: an appropriate work-to-rest ratio, balance in work and play, balance in self-study and intimacy with others. In whatever yoga pose you are in, or in whatever condition you are challenged with in life, the key is to establish balance.

Balance also helps you realign to the present moment, because balance itself is in the state of the present—the here and now. When you are deeply concentrating, extending your awareness through the body to maintain balance, you are living in the present moment. When the body and mind are stable and balanced, there is no past and no future. There is only the perfect balance and equilibrium of the present moment. The tendency of the mind is to project you into the future, as it plans, worries, and wonders. Your memory takes you into the past, where it revisits, replays, regrets, and rehashes. However, when your mind evenly spreads through the body, as is necessary during the balancing poses of yoga, you remain rooted in the present moment. In these initially brief glimpses of absolute present moment awareness, the mind can be trained to return to the state of bliss for a more regular and sustained length of time.

LIGHTNESS

When an Olympic lifting technique or kettlebell technique is done correctly, there is a sensation of lightness in the trajectory of the weight. As with yoga, the movements of the body should be smooth, and a feeling of lightness, openness, and freedom should be cultivated in the mind. The energy of worry and regret, taking place in the past or future, is heavy and burdensome for the mind. However, the light feelings associated with joy and happiness are easy on the mind. By extending a feeling of lightness through the body, the same feeling can be extended through the mind, and the correlating feelings of happiness, faithfulness, and courage can be expressed. Lightness is expressed in all yoga poses by extending from the core outward. The opposite of extension in yoga is slouching, which acts on the body like a depressant. The primary function of the spine in yoga is to keep the mind sharp, alert, and aware. To achieve this, in all yoga poses, and in life, the spine must reach up to the heavens. The openness of the spine and upright posture of the body achieved through yoga results in a sense of physical and mental lightness—we begin to "feel lighter" while simultaneously radiating more light in our life.

EXTENSION

The goal of the yoga pose is to extend from the core of your being through the extremities and periphery of your body. From your head to your heels, establish your center, and from this center, extend and expand in all directions. To stretch in yoga means to extend and expand at the same time, which brings space. The resulting space brings freedom in the joints and muscles of the body and freedom for creativity in the mind. Extension in yoga also teaches how to establish fullness in the pose, and the fullness of each pose teaches how to be full in whatever you are doing in your life.

PRESENCE

The manner in which you are relating to the body and breath in a yoga pose is the manner in which you are relating to life. Each yoga pose is a micro-lesson for life. The pose will continue to provide an opportunity to learn a lesson, until the lesson is learned. Similarly, life will continue to give you an opportunity to learn a lesson in increasing volume and intensity, until the lesson is learned.

There are three keys to developing presence in yoga. Think of these three master keys as complementary to each other—each arising in a harmonious manner in a never-ending process of present-moment awareness.

1. Continually align and realign to the present moment.
2. Practice a state of non-reaction to the nature of the present moment. Release the tendency of the mind to want to establish control or wish things were different than they are.
3. Cultivate compassion for the present moment. View things as happening *for* you, not *to* you. Have compassion for the present moment because the universe is providing you an opportunity to grow.

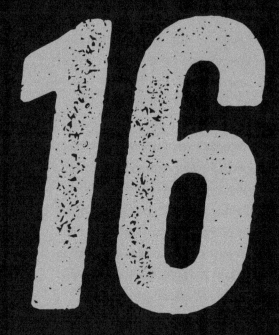

16

SATVANA: FIREBREATHER YOGA

SATVANA YOGA

IN YOGA, there is no shortage of versions and interpretations. While the poses—the operating language of yoga—are generally the same, yoga teachers have created different forms of the practice to serve different people, different needs, and different goals.

My own version of yoga, designed to work within the Firebreather Fitness program, is called Satvana yoga. In Satvana yoga, our body of practice is referred to as "Satvanaga." This term comes from the Sanskrit word "Satvana," which means "warrior," and is combined with the Sanskrit word "yoga," which means "union."

On a physical level, Satvana yoga brings deep awareness in understanding how the body moves in space and time. Through dedicated practice, a student's senses turn inward and develop the ability to listen and feel with refined skill and sensitivity. Practitioners have a deepened sense of intuition and awareness. Furthermore, the inner strength that practitioners develop spills over into physical pursuits, improving quality of movement, virtuosity, and gracefulness.

On an internal level, Satvana yoga connects students with their higher self, life purpose, and the spiritual realm.

On www.firebreatherfitness.org, you'll find many yoga resources, including videos that you can follow to learn the routines as I teach them in my studio. But the purpose of this book is simply to give you some tools to begin and get traction with a small but complete program, one that respects that you probably have little time to spare in the first place.

I have gained tremendous benefits from practicing yoga just 15 minutes per day, with an extended period on weekends. But even if you have less time, you'll gain an immense amount if you are consistent.

Over the years, I have grown to greatly appreciate the principle of quality over quantity. When it comes to practicing yoga, nothing could be more true. Furthermore, it is important to understand the word "practice" in relation to "practicing yoga." When you are engaged in the physical workouts associated with the Firebreather Fitness plan, you are *training*. While maintaining adherence to range of motion and technique, you are blasting through workouts as fast as possible, reaping the benefits of relative intensity. However, with yoga, I want you to focus on turning your attention inward to the more subtle energy systems within your body. By "practicing yoga" I ask you to move beyond the physical nature of exercise, and into the mental and spiritual realm. Because every movement in yoga is associated with a corresponding breath, the practice of yoga "yokes" you to the present moment. When the mind wanders, simply return to the breath and the next movement of your body. In this context, you are practicing present-moment awareness and benefiting from the experience of contentment, peace, and tranquility.

Perform the Satvana series on the following pages, either as a warm-up for your day's workout or as part of your morning wake-up routine. In the 21-day plans, I have inserted the series into the programs every fourth day, as part of your active rest and recovery. On these days, feel free to move through this series up to five times, holding each pose for up to four breaths.

These yoga poses should be practiced slowly, with attention to detail, fluidity, gracefulness, and ease. Do not exert unnecessary force in any pose. Rather, focus on striking a balance between effort and ease. Move between poses according to your own level of strength, flexibility, and capacity. Awareness, concentration, and evenness of breath are more important

Satvana yoga connects students with their higher self, life purpose, and the spiritual realm.

than how a pose looks. Follow the pattern of breath sequencing that I teach as you move into and out of each pose. If you wish to hold a pose for an extended period of time, move into the pose through the breath sequence, then breathe naturally while holding the pose. Always inhale and exhale through the nostrils unless specified differently. The breath should be smooth, slow, and deep, and should originate in the lower abdomen, fill the lungs completely, and rise into the shoulders and head. The movement of the body should complement the breath, and in this context, the breath should lead the body. Following your practice of yoga, finish with a relaxing pose, either lying completely still on your back or seated comfortably, with the back straight and eyes closed.

I have described the yoga poses in a manner that you can understand the starting position of each pose, and their relationship together. Keep in mind, however, each pose could be practiced in isolation.

SUN SALUTATION

>> Begin your practice with a standing sun salutation.

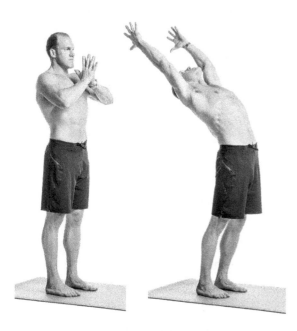

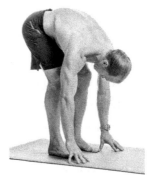

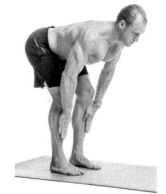

1 Start in mountain pose, with palms together over heart. Feet are hip-width apart and pointing forward. Legs are fully extended, and crown of head reaches for the sky. Eyes are open with a soft gaze. Take four slow deep breaths. This is a pose of deep reverence for the great spirit within you, with recognition and awareness the spirit within you is also within everyone else.

2 At the beginning of your fifth inhalation, sweep arms overhead and then behind you, lifting heart toward the sky. Come into a backbend that is comfortable for you, or simply raise arms straight overhead, bringing gaze to the sky. Take four deep breaths.

3 At the bottom of the fourth exhalation, gracefully arc arms to the ground, allowing the breath to lead the body. Come into a forward fold. Draw belly into spine and engage quadriceps and abdominal muscles. Legs can be slightly bent to aid the pose. Distribute weight evenly through feet. Take four deep breaths.

4 At the beginning of the fifth inhalation, lengthen the spine by pressing palms against shin bones. Back should be arched, similar to the spinal alignment created in a deadlift. Head maintains a clean line of energy through spine. Gaze is soft. Take four deep breaths.

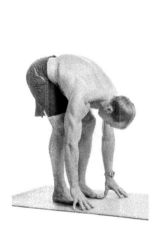 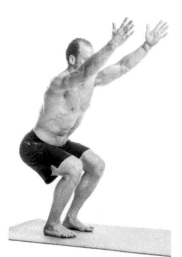 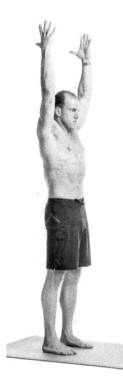

5 At the bottom of the fourth exhalation, return into forward fold, allowing the breath to lead the body. Take four deep breaths.

6 At the end of the fourth exhalation, bend knees and drop hips, while inhaling and extending arms forward, above shoulder height, and come into chair pose. Take four deep breaths.

7 At the beginning of your fifth inhalation, extend evenly through legs, and return to mountain pose. Take four deep breaths.

DOWNWARD DOG

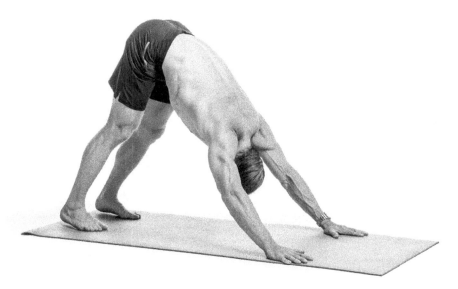

>> In this pose, your body creates an inverted V position. Hands are placed just outside shoulders with fingers spread, and palms of hands press evenly through the ground. Quadriceps are engaged, and scapula draws down the spine. Heels are either on the floor or energetically moving in that direction. The priority in the pose is an extended and straight back; allow the legs to slightly bend if necessary. Head is in alignment with spine.

POINTS OF PERFORMANCE

Focus on actively pressing through the mat with hands and feet, while lifting hips toward the sky. Remain strong through the side body, and focus on feeling the breath move upward through the body.

WARRIOR I

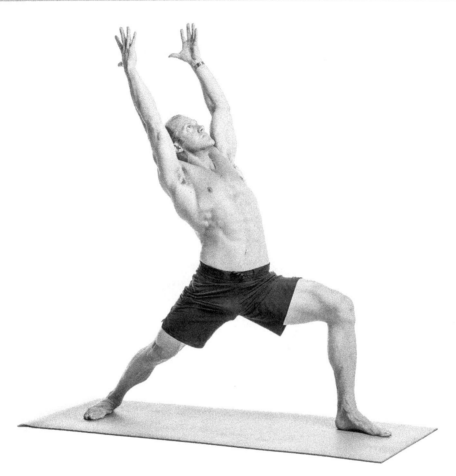

>> Establish a stable base, with feet approximately 3 to 4 feet apart, measured from heel to heel. Lead foot is at a 90-degree angle, with lead knee stacked over lead foot. The back foot and ankle form an angle of 45 degrees. Rotate pelvis down and in, drawing belly button in toward the spine. Expand through the muscles along the sides of your abdomen and lats, and keep rib cage drawn in. Extend your arms alongside your head, sending energy out through the tips of the fingers. Your gaze is steady and focused toward the sky, and breath evenly fills the body.

POINTS OF PERFORMANCE

This is the pose of a warrior; the physical quality of the pose should match its emotional and energetic intention: courage, service, strength, resolve. Draw energy in through the feet, gather energy in the core, and then shine out through the hands. Hug skin to muscle, and muscle to bone.

WARRIOR II

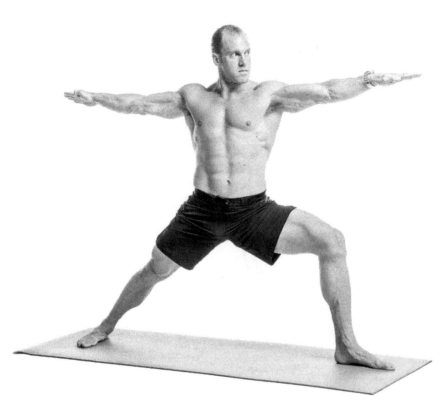

As in Warrior I, position feet approximately 3 to 4 feet apart, with heels in alignment or slightly offset. Lead foot is at a 90-degree angle, with shin vertical and knee stacked over ankle. Back foot is at 45 degrees. Hips are open and evenly stacked over the floor. The back leg is in extension, and the knife-edge portion of back foot presses through the mat. Torso is upright and chest is open, with shoulders evenly stacked over hips. Arms are extended and stacked over legs. Energy is drawn up through feet and shines through fingertips. Keep pelvis tucked and back straight, and draw belly button in toward the spine. Latissimus muscles are active and expand with every breath.

POINTS OF PERFORMANCE

This pose's intention is to cultivate a warrior's determination for advancement, while being content in the present moment. Focus on balancing effort with ease, finding a sweet spot that evenly matches strength with grace.

WARRIOR III

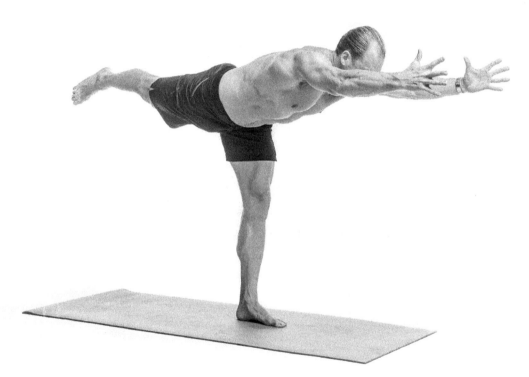

>> From Warrior II, shift weight onto forward leg. Root forward foot into the ground, and extend the leg. A slight bend in the forward leg is OK—energetically work toward extension. Extend rear leg up behind you and keep it active. Keep balancing leg rooted and strong. Extend arms to front of mat, creating a clean line of energy from heel of extended leg, through spine, and shining out through the fingers.

POINTS OF PERFORMANCE

This is the most challenging warrior pose. It is a balancing pose, which helps to achieve structural integration in the body, mental stability, and focused attention. Balancing the body can help achieve mental and emotional balance.

EXALTED WARRIOR

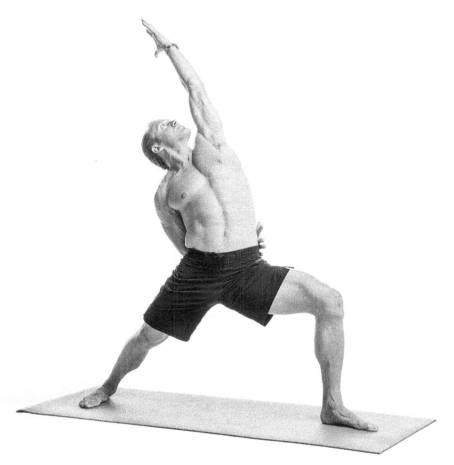

⟫ Lead hand moves up and back as you inhale, opening into a backbend. Your rear hand gently draws to rear leg or wraps behind low back. Gaze is drawn up over fingers of the lead hand.

POINTS OF PERFORMANCE
Exalted Warrior offers the heart and mind up into a backbend, seeking the higher self. Lead hand continues to reach higher and higher. The strength of the spine maintains the backbend.

EXTENDED SIDE ANGLE

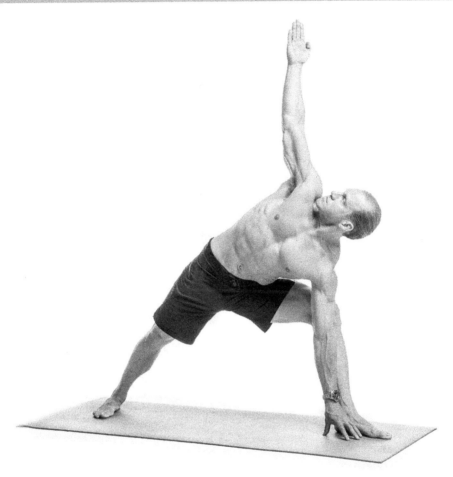

From Exalted Warrior, leading arm is placed alongside inner thigh and maintains contact during pose. Lead hand is placed alongside lead foot. Right hip draws back and stacks over left hip, while right shoulder simultaneously draws back and stacks over left shoulder. Chest is open, and a clean line of energy runs from the leading hand, through chest and heart, and shines through extended hand.

POINTS OF PERFORMANCE

Imagine in this pose your body is suspended between two sheets of glass. Seen from the front, your body should be evenly stacked on top of itself, taking up only as much space as your stacked hips. Keep the upward hip lifting during the pose, and feel into the clean line of energy from back foot, through rear leg, and through extended side body.

REVERSE TRIANGLE

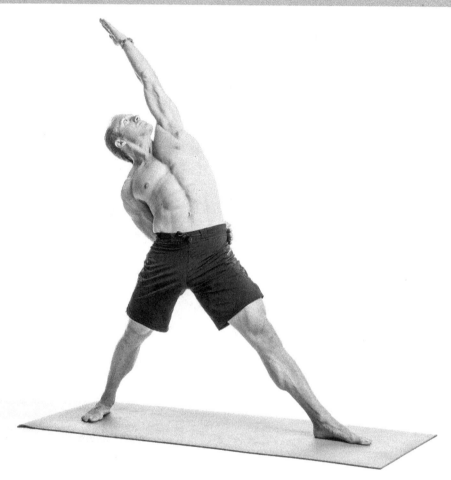

From Extended Side Angle, both legs come into complete extension. The toes of the lead leg are facing forward, and the back foot is at a 45-degree angle. The heels are either in alignment, or the heel of the lead leg intersects arch of back foot. The lead arm points toward the heavens, and the support arm is gently placed against the back leg, or wrapped behind the back. A clean line of energy runs from lead foot, through lead leg, hip, and side body, and shines through lead arm.

POINTS OF PERFORMANCE

Press both feet through the mat, drawing energy in from the earth, and shining that energy into the sky through the extended arm. Breath is open and expansive, and gaze is up.

Forge an indomitable mind, body, and spirit.

Apply character traits learned on the mat to life:

Purity – Truthfulness – Peacefulness – Contentment –

Austerity – Surrender – Willpower and *Namaste*.

Be Humble.

Encourage others.

SATVANA SERIES

After practicing each of the poses in isolation, it's time to connect breath, mind, and body through a continual flow.

1 Complete four standing Sun Salutations.

2 At the completion of fourth round, allow the breath to lead the body, and come into a forward fold. From a forward fold, walk hands forward into Downward Dog. Take four deep breaths.

3 At the bottom of the fourth breath, step left foot forward, and then inhale and sweep arms overhead, coming into Warrior I. Rear leg will rotate into position as arms extend. Hold for four deep breaths.

4 At the bottom of the fourth breath, transition into Warrior II. Hold for four deep breaths.

5 From Warrior II, move into Warrior III by exhaling and shifting weight forward onto left foot, simultaneously extending back leg into the air. Reach hands forward, bringing body weight onto left leg. Hold for four deep breaths.

6 At the bottom of the fourth breath, step right leg gently to mat, returning to the lower body position of Warrior II, while simultaneously extending left arm into the air and wrapping right arm around low back. Hold Exalted Warrior for four deep breaths.

7 At the bottom of the fourth breath, flow directly into Extended Side Angle pose. Allow the breath to lead the body. Hold for four deep breaths.

8 At the beginning of the fifth inhalation, extend through left leg, and sweep left arm overhead, coming into Reverse Triangle pose. Hold for four deep breaths.

9 Following this sequence, step right leg forward and return to Mountain pose, with hands at heart center. Then complete one Sun Salutation, flowing from forward fold into the warrior sequence on the opposite side of the body.

For the complete Satvana yoga series, visit www.firebreatherfitness.org and go through it with me on video.

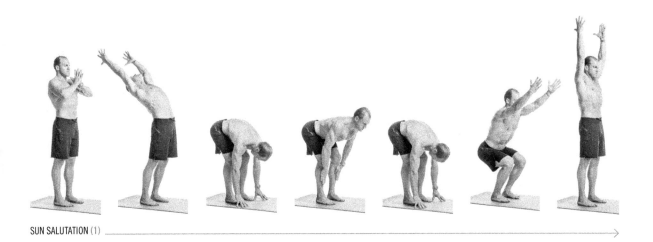

SUN SALUTATION (1) ——→

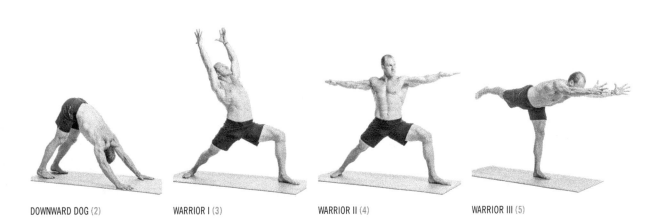

DOWNWARD DOG (2)   WARRIOR I (3)   WARRIOR II (4)   WARRIOR III (5)

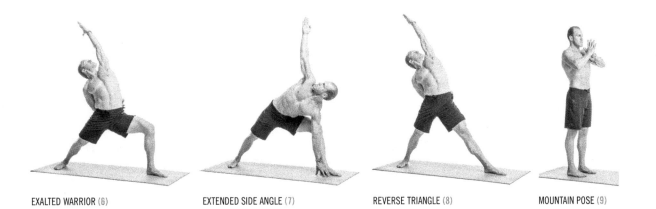

EXALTED WARRIOR (6)   EXTENDED SIDE ANGLE (7)   REVERSE TRIANGLE (8)   MOUNTAIN POSE (9)

PLANS

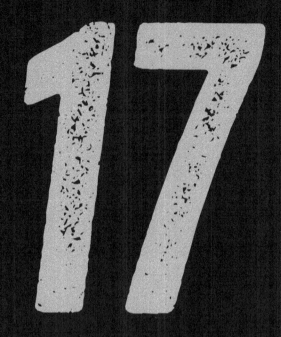

FIREBREATHER FITNESS:
21-DAY PLANS

IT'S TIME TO START BREATHING FIRE.

The following are your integrated training plans. These comprehensive 21-day plans integrate your mind, body, and spirit for optimal performance and lasting results.

The plans include several mind and spirit practices to complement your daily physical workouts. Think of these practices in a linear fashion, like a handrail that is leading you through your day. First words and meditation are terrific ways to begin each morning. These practices set you on the road to success and help you connect with your higher self, your unique purpose in life, and with God (or Spirit, the Universe, etc.). Box breathing and affirmations help focus your energy and willpower for your workout of the day. Then, during the workout, discipline yourself to pay attention to your breathing and continue to repeat your positive mantras and affirmations. When the going gets tough, refocus yourself by committing to your purpose, and embrace the work set before you. You are developing the Firebreather mind-set: being optimistic even in the face of great challenge. In the evening, adopt a habit of journaling, recording impressions of how the process is evolving (see "Journaling" sidebar, page 231). Reflect on your biggest accomplishments of the day, and write three things you are grateful for. In 21 days, you will see solid progress in your physical, mental, and spiritual fitness.

If you have doubts about the value of incorporating mental and spiritual practices into your physical fitness program, I say this: Give it your best shot over the 21-day period. Support it with a Zone nutrition program (see Chapter 6). By the time the 21 days are up, I believe you will notice a profound effect on how you view yourself and what you're capable of in life. With the majority of athletes I coach, the consensus is that the progress made mentally, emotionally, and spiritually always surpasses the gains made physically. And what is even more exciting is that the physical gains made are big!

As for which program to choose, I recommend everyone start with the beginner program. This gives you a chance to learn the Firebreather Fitness methodology. Each level builds progressively upon the last. An advanced athlete who starts with the beginner program and feels it is too easy can bypass the intermediate plan and move directly and safely to the advanced program. Only advance to the next level of the program if you are able to complete all workouts with the prescribed weights, repetitions, and percentage requirements. Keep in mind that as your strength and physical capacity increase, each program will become more challenging. Therefore, even the beginner program, if repeated continually over a year, will get progressively more challenging. This is the beauty of the Firebreather Fitness program: It's a living and breathing program that adapts to your conditioning level.

Note that many of the weight lifting skills take place after your gymnastic conditioning. This is crucial to the philosophy of the Firebreather, which involves maintaining strength at a high heart rate. Just ask any military operator or law-enforcement officer, and he or she will confirm that in critical moments when you need your strength, you will need it at a high heart rate. Your training should reflect and prepare you for the demands of life!

Also, note that rather than prescribing a specific weight to utilize on the barbell skills, you are training at a percentage of your relative strength. This specific percentage, unique to each level of the 21-day plan, will be assigned in the workouts. This aspect of the Firebreather Fitness plan allows a lifetime of continued adaptation, challenge, and growth.

The plan includes your physical workouts along with a basic set of rituals to weave into your day: first words, meditation, box breathing, and positive affirmations.

If you are new to these movements and practices, you may at first feel overwhelmed or a little intimidated. But don't think about the 21-day plan as a whole. The program offers an excellent opportunity to practice the power of microgoals. Commit to the big goal of completing the plan, and then narrow your focus to the task list for Day One. Make that your universe! This way, all you have to focus on is completing a small set of tasks during the course of a single day. The discipline to take life one moment at a time, and to remain aware and committed to living in the present, is the Firebreather way and the skill of a warrior. Therefore, take these workouts and practices one day at a time, trusting in the compound effect and long-term benefit the program will provide.

21-DAY BEGINNER PLAN

The 21-day beginner plan is designed to develop your confidence, technique, and capacity in a combined weight lifting and gymnastic conditioning program, and to introduce you to the concepts of an integrated and holistic approach to fitness.

DAY 1	DAY 2	DAY 3
4 rounds of box breathing	*4 rounds of box breathing*	*4 rounds of box breathing*
5 min. of meditation	*5 min. of meditation*	*5 min. of meditation*
Eyes closed: 10 reps of mantra or affirmation	*Eyes closed: 10 reps of mantra or affirmation*	*Eyes closed: 10 reps of mantra or affirmation*
First words	*First words*	*First words*
BASELINE WORKOUT	**AMRAP MASH-UP TEST #1**	Thruster, 5,3,1,1,1 reps (work up to a 1RM)
AMRAP in 10:00 of:	AMRAP in 1:00 of jump rope	Rest 2:00 and find your 30% threshold of 1RM
30 squats	Rest 1:00	
20 push-ups		4 rounds for time:
10 pull-ups (use a band if necessary, or ring row)	AMRAP in 1:00 of kettlebell swing (men: 35 lb. / women: 25 lb.)	Run 400m (or row 400m)
From 10:00 to 15:00:	Rest 2:00 and determine your 30% threshold	10 ring rows
Find your 1 rep max power clean		Thruster, 5 reps (30% 1RM)
	EMOM for 10:00 (5 rounds of each):	
	Odd min. = 30% threshold for jump rope	
	Even min. = 30% threshold for kettlebell swing	

TERMINOLOGY

Box breathing = 4-count breathing exercise (see page 176)
Mantra or affirmation = your personal belief statement (see page 181)
First words = the warrior practice of mindful speaking (see page 146)
AMRAP = as many rounds (or reps) as possible

Threshold = your 100% max effort
EMOM = every minute on the minute
RM = 1 rep max effort

DAY 4

4 rounds of box breathing

5 min. of meditation

Eyes closed: 10 reps of mantra or affirmation

First words

Fitness Outside the Box (walk, run, hike, swim, surf, play!)

Spend 15:00 practicing your overhead squat and Satvana yoga series

DAY 5

4 rounds of box breathing

5 min. of meditation

Eyes closed: 10 reps of mantra or affirmation

First words

AMRAP MASH-UP TEST #2

AMRAP in 1:00 of wall ball (men: 20 lb., 10 ft. / women: 14 lb., 8ft.)

Rest 1:00

AMRAP in 1:00 of pull-up (use a band if necessary)

Rest 2:00 and determine your 30% threshold

EMOM for 12:00 (6 rounds of each):

Odd min. = 30% threshold for wall ball

Even min. = 30% threshold for pull-up

DAY 6

4 rounds of box breathing

5 min. of meditation

Eyes closed: 10 reps of mantra or affirmation

First words

AMRAP MASH-UP TEST #3

AMRAP in 1:00 of knees-to-elbow

Rest 1:00

AMRAP in 1:00 of box jump (men: 20 in. / women: 16 in.)

Rest 1:00

AMRAP in 1:00 of push-up

Rest 2:00 and determine your 40% threshold

Every 3 min. for 12:00 (4 rounds each):

Min. 1 = 40% threshold for knees-to-elbow

Min. 2 = 40% threshold for box jump

Min. 3 = 40% threshold for push-up

DAY 7

4 rounds of box breathing

5 min. of meditation

Eyes closed: 10 reps of mantra or affirmation

First words

Bench press, 5,3,1,1,1 reps (work up to 1RM bench press)

Back squat, 5,3,1,1,1 reps (work up to a 1RM squat)

Rest 2:00 and determine 30% of 1RM bench and 1RM squat

4 rounds for time:

Run 400m (or row 400m)

Back squat, 9 reps (30% 1RM)

Bench press, 6 reps (30% 1RM)

DAY 8	DAY 9	DAY 10	DAY 11
4 rounds of box breathing	*4 rounds of box breathing*	*4 rounds of box breathing*	*4 rounds of box breathing*
5 min. of meditation	*5 min. of meditation*	*5 min. of meditation*	*5 min. of meditation*
Eyes closed: 10 reps of mantra or affirmation	*Eyes closed: 10 reps of mantra or affirmation*	*Eyes closed: 10 reps of mantra or affirmation*	*Eyes closed: 10 reps of mantra or affirmation*
First words	*First words*	*First words*	*First words*

DAY 8	DAY 9	DAY 10	DAY 11
Fitness Outside the Box (walk, run, hike, swim, surf, play!) Spend 15:00 practicing Satvana yoga and overhead squat	**AMRAP MASH-UP EVOLUTION #1 (FORMERLY TEST #1)** EMOM for 10:00 (5 rounds of each): Odd min. = 40% threshold for jump rope Even min. = 40% threshold for kettlebell swing	On a 10:00 running clock: Power clean, 30 reps (30% 1RM) 10 burpees Power clean, AMRAP (30% 1RM) *Note: For this workout, your "score" is your final set of power cleans.*	**AMRAP MASH-UP EVOLUTION #2 (FORMERLY TEST #2)** EMOM for 10:00 (5 rounds of each): Odd min. = 40% threshold for wall ball Even min. = 40% threshold for pull-up

DAY 12

4 rounds of box breathing

5 min. of meditation

Eyes closed: 10 reps of mantra or affirmation

First words

Fitness Outside the Box (walk, run, hike, swim, surf, play!)

Complete the full Satvana yoga series

DAY 13

4 rounds of box breathing

5 min. of meditation

Eyes closed: 10 reps of mantra or affirmation

First words

AMRAP MASH-UP EVOLUTION #3 (FORMERLY TEST #3)

Every 3 min. for 15:00 (5 rounds each):

Min. 1 = 40% threshold for knees-to-elbow

Min. 2 = 40% threshold for box jump (men: 20 in. / women: 16 in.)

Min. 3 = 40% threshold for push-up

DAY 14

4 rounds of box breathing

5 minutes of meditation

Eyes closed: 10 repetitions of mantra or affirmation

First words

Shoulder press, 5,3,1,1,1 reps (establish a 1RM)

Rest 2:00 and determine 30% of your 1RM press

4 rounds for time:

Push press, 15 reps (30% 1RM)

30 squats

10 pull-ups (or ring rows)

Note: Although the 1RM that you will establish is your press, in the workout, utilize the push press.

DAY 15

4 rounds of box breathing

5 min. of meditation

Eyes closed: 10 reps of mantra or affirmation

First words

AMRAP MASH-UP EVOLUTION #1 (FORMERLY TEST #1)

EMOM for 12:00 (6 rounds of each):

Odd min. = 40% threshold for jump rope

Even min. = 40% threshold for kettlebell swing (men: 35 lb. / women: 25 lb.)

21-DAY BEGINNER PLAN (Continued)

DAY 16

4 rounds of box breathing

5 min. of meditation

Eyes closed: 10 reps of mantra or affirmation

First words

Fitness Outside the Box (walk, run, hike, swim, surf, play!)

Spend 10:00 practicing your overhead squat and 5 rounds of Satvana yoga sun salutation

DAY 17

4 rounds of box breathing

5 min. of meditation

Eyes closed: 10 reps of mantra or affirmation

First words

AMRAP in 15:00 of:

Run 400m (or row 400m)

10 burpees

Thruster, 5 reps (30% 1RM)

DAY 18

4 rounds of box breathing

5 min. of meditation

Eyes closed: 10 reps of mantra or affirmation

First words

---

3 rounds for time:

Jump rope, 100 reps

Kettlebell swing, 20 reps (men: 35 lb. / women: 25 lb.)

10 ring rows

DAY 19

4 rounds of box breathing

5 min. of meditation

Eyes closed: 10 reps of mantra or affirmation

First words

AMRAP in 10:00 of the rep scheme below:

Power clean, 3 reps (30% 1RM)

Knees-to-elbow, 3 reps

Power clean, 6 reps

Knees-to-elbow, 6 reps

Power clean, 9 reps

Knees-to-elbow, 9 reps

Power clean, 12 reps

Knees-to-elbow, 12 reps

Power clean, 15 reps

Knees-to-elbow, 15 reps

This is a timed workout. If you complete the round of 15, go on to 18. If you complete 18, go on to 21, etc.

DAY 20

4 rounds of box breathing

5 min. of meditation

Eyes closed: 10 reps of mantra or affirmation

First words

Fitness Outside the Box (walk, run, hike, swim, surf, play!)

Complete the full Satvana yoga series and spend 10:00 practicing your overhead squat

DAY 21

4 rounds of box breathing

5 min. of meditation

Eyes closed: 10 reps of mantra or affirmation

First words

BASELINE WORKOUT RETEST

AMRAP in 10:00 of:

30 squats

20 push-ups

10 pull-ups
(use a band if necessary)

From 10:00 to 15:00:

Find your 1 rep max power clean

Congratulations! You've just created an amazing amount of momentum in your life, and begun the process of integrating your mind, body, and spirit. Your 21-day challenge can now become a measurable and repeatable fitness plan. Here is how it works:

Go back to AMRAP Mash-Up Tests 1, 2, and 3, and retest your AMRAP potential. You will be happy to see an improvement in your capacity. Then, repeat the remaining workouts, recalculating your threshold accordingly. You will follow the same protocol for your weight lifting workouts. Every three months, take a week off: Just practice yoga and enjoy Fitness Outside the Box. When you are able to meet these workouts "as prescribed," or without modifications, then move on to the more challenging intermediate Firebreather plan.

Be creative. Have fun!

21-DAY INTERMEDIATE PLAN

The 21-day intermediate Firebreather Fitness plan builds on the beginner plan and helps prepare you for the supercharged advanced plan. Note that many of the weight lifting skills take place after your gymnastic conditioning. This is crucial to the philosophy of the Firebreather, which is maintaining strength at a high heart rate.

DAY 1	DAY 2	DAY 3
4 rounds of box breathing	*4 rounds of box breathing*	*4 rounds of box breathing*
10 min. of meditation	*10 min. of meditation*	*10 min. of meditation*
Eyes closed: 10 reps of mantra or affirmation	*Eyes closed: 10 reps of mantra or affirmation*	*Eyes closed: 10 reps of mantra or affirmation*
First words	*First words*	*First words*

DAY 1	DAY 2	DAY 3
BASELINE WORKOUT	**AMRAP MASH-UP TEST #1**	Thruster, 5,3,1,1,1 reps (work up to a 1RM weight)
AMRAP in 10:00 of:	AMRAP in 1:00 of jump rope (double under)	Rest 2:00 and find your 50% threshold of 1RM
50 squats	Rest 1:00	
30 push-ups		4 rounds for time:
10 pull-ups	AMRAP in 1:00 of kettlebell swing (men: 35 lb. / women: 25 lb.)	Run 400m (or row 400m)
From 10:00 to 15:00:	Rest 2:00 and determine your 40% threshold	10 burpees
Find your 1 rep max power clean		Thruster, 5 reps (50% 1RM)
	EMOM for 12:00 (6 rounds of each):	
	Odd min. = 40% threshold for jump rope (double under)	
	Even min. = 40% threshold for kettlebell swing	

TERMINOLOGY

Box breathing = 4-count breathing exercise (see page 176)

Mantra or affirmation = your personal belief statement (see page 181)

First words = the warrior practice of mindful speaking (see page 146)

AMRAP = as many rounds (or reps) as possible

Threshold = your 100% max effort

EMOM = every minute on the minute

RM = 1 rep max effort

DAY 4

4 rounds of box breathing

10 min. of meditation

Eyes closed: 10 reps of mantra or affirmation

First words

Fitness Outside the Box (walk, run, hike, swim, surf, play!)

Spend 15:00 practicing your overhead squat and Satvana yoga series

DAY 5

4 rounds of box breathing

10 min. of meditation

Eyes closed: 10 reps of mantra or affirmation

First words

AMRAP MASH-UP TEST #2

AMRAP in 1:00 of wall ball (men: 20 lb., 10 ft. / women: 14 lb., 8 ft.)

Rest 1:00

AMRAP in 1:00 of pull-up

Rest 2:00 and determine your 40% threshold

EMOM for 10:00 (5 rounds of each):

Odd min. = 40% threshold for wall ball

Even min. = 40% threshold for pull-up

DAY 6

4 rounds of box breathing

10 min. of meditation

Eyes closed: 10 reps of mantra or affirmation

First words

AMRAP MASH-UP TEST #3

AMRAP in 1:00 of toes-to-bar

Rest 1:00

AMRAP in 1:00 of box jumps (men: 24 in. / women: 20 in.)

Rest 1:00

AMRAP in 1:00 of push-ups

Rest 2:00 and determine your 40% threshold

Every 3 min. for 15:00 (5 rounds each):

Min. 1 = 40% threshold for toes-to-bar

Min. 2 = 40% threshold for box jumps

Min. 3 = 40% threshold for push-ups

DAY 7

4 rounds of box breathing

10 min. of meditation

Eyes closed: 10 reps of mantra or affirmation

First words

Bench press, 5,3,1,1,1 reps (work up to a 1RM bench press)

Back squat, 5,3,1,1,1 reps (work up to a 1RM squat)

Rest 2:00 and determine 50% of 1RM bench and 1RM squat

4 rounds for time:

Run 400m (or row 400m)

Back squat, 12 reps (50% 1RM)

Bench press, 9 reps (50% 1RM)

10 pull-ups

21-DAY INTERMEDIATE PLAN *(Continued)*

DAY 8

4 rounds of box breathing

10 min. of meditation

Eyes closed: 10 reps of mantra or affirmation

First words

Fitness Outside the Box (walk, run, hike, swim, surf, play!)

Spend 15:00 on Satvana yoga and practicing your overhead squat

DAY 9

4 rounds of box breathing

10 min. of meditation

Eyes closed: 10 reps of mantra or affirmation

First words

AMRAP MASH-UP EVOLUTION #1 (FORMERLY TEST #1)

EMOM for 12:00 (6 rounds of each):

Odd min. = 50% threshold for jump rope (double under)

Even min. = 50% threshold for kettlebell swing

DAY 10

4 rounds of box breathing

10 min. of meditation

Eyes closed: 10 reps of mantra or affirmation

First words

Clean and jerk, 5,3,1,1,1 reps (work up to a 1RM weight)

Rest 2:00 and find your 50% threshold of 1RM

On a 10:00 running clock:

Clean and jerk, 30 reps (50% 1RM)

Burpee and pull-up, 20 reps

Clean and jerk, AMRAP (50% 1RM)

Note: For this workout, your "score" is your final set of clean and jerks. A "burpee and pull-up" means a full range of motion burpee, then as you jump into the air, instead of clapping your hands, grab the pull-up bar, and complete a pull-up. Come off the bar, and repeat for the prescribed repetitions.

DAY 11

4 rounds of box breathing

10 min. of meditation

Eyes closed: 10 reps of mantra or affirmation

First words

AMRAP MASH-UP EVOLUTION #2 (FORMERLY TEST #2)

EMOM for 12:00 (6 rounds of each):

Odd min. = 50% threshold for wall ball

Even min. = 50% threshold for pull-up

DAY 12

4 rounds of box breathing

10 min. of meditation

Eyes closed: 10 reps of mantra or affirmation

First words

Fitness Outside the Box (walk, run, hike, swim, surf, play!)

Complete the full Satvana yoga series

DAY 13

4 rounds of box breathing

10 min. of meditation

Eyes closed: 10 reps of mantra or affirmation

First words

AMRAP MASH-UP EVOLUTION #3 (FORMERLY TEST #3)

Every 3 min. for 15:00 (5 rounds each):

Min. 1 = 50% threshold for toes-to-bar

Min. 2 = 50% threshold for box jump (men: 24 in. / women: 20 in.)

Min. 3 = 50% threshold for push-up

DAY 14

4 rounds of box breathing

10 min. of meditation

Eyes closed: 10 reps of mantra or affirmation

First words

Shoulder press, 5,3,1,1,1 reps (establish a 1RM)

Rest 2:00 and determine 50% of your 1RM press

4 rounds for time:

Run 400m (or row 400m)

Push press, 15 reps (50% 1RM)

20 weighted alternating lunges, 10 each leg (men: 25 lb. / women: 15 lb.)

Note: Although the 1RM that you will establish is your press, in the workout, utilize the push press.

DAY 15

4 rounds of box breathing

10 min. of meditation

Eyes closed: 10 reps of mantra or affirmation

First words

AMRAP MASH-UP EVOLUTION #1 (FORMERLY TEST #1)

EMOM for 10:00 (5 rounds of each):

Odd min. = 60% threshold for double under

Even min. = 60% threshold for kettlebell swing (men: 35 lb. / women: 25 lb.)

DAY 16

4 rounds of box breathing

10 min. of meditation

Eyes closed: 10 reps of mantra or affirmation

First words

Fitness Outside the Box (walk, run, hike, swim, surf, play!)

Spend 10:00 practicing your overhead squat and 10 rounds of Satvana yoga sun salutation

DAY 17

4 rounds of box breathing

10 min. of meditation

Eyes closed: 10 reps of mantra or affirmation

First words

AMRAP in 20:00 of:

Run 400m (or row 400m)

10 burpees

Thruster, 5 reps (60% 1RM)

DAY 18

4 rounds of box breathing

10 min. of meditation

Eyes closed: 10 reps of mantra or affirmation

First words

Deadlift, 5,3,1,1,1 reps (establish a 1RM)

Rest 4:00 and determine 40% 1RM deadlift

For time:

Deadlift, 21 reps (40% 1RM)

Bar dip, 21 reps

Deadlift, 15 reps

Bar dip, 15 reps

Deadlift, 9 reps

Bar dip, 9 reps

DAY 19

4 rounds of box breathing

10 min. of meditation

Eyes closed: 10 reps of mantra or affirmation

First words

AMRAP MASH-UP EVOLUTION #3 (FORMERLY TEST #3)

Every 3 min. for 15:00 (5 rounds each):

Min. 1 = 60% threshold for toes-to-bar

Min. 2 = 60% threshold for box jump (men: 24 in. / women: 20 in.)

Min. 3 = 60% threshold for push-up

DAY 20

4 rounds of box breathing

10 min. of meditation

Eyes closed: 10 reps of mantra or affirmation

First words

Fitness Outside the Box (walk, run, hike, swim, surf, play!)

Complete the full Satvana yoga series and spend 10:00 practicing your overhead squat

DAY 21

4 rounds of box breathing

10 min. of meditation

Eyes closed: 10 reps of mantra or affirmation

First words

BASELINE WORKOUT RETEST

AMRAP in 10:00 of:

50 squats

30 push-ups

10 pull-ups

From 10:00 to 15:00:

Find your 1 rep max power clean

Just like with the beginner plan, this 21-day challenge can now become a measurable and repeatable fitness plan. Here is how it works:

Go back to AMRAP Mash-Up Tests 1, 2, and 3, and retest your AMRAP potential. You will be happy to see an improvement in your capacity. Then, repeat the remaining workouts, recalculating your threshold accordingly. You will follow the same protocol for your weight lifting workouts. Every three months, take a week off and just practice yoga, and enjoy Fitness Outside the Box. When you are able to meet these workouts as prescribed, or without modifications, then move on to the supercharged advanced Firebreather plan!

21-DAY ADVANCED PLAN

The 21-day advanced Firebreather Fitness plan is a life-changing, momentum creating, and holistically integrated program designed to propel you into the best shape of your life. Stay the course, believe in yourself, and as my friend Mark Divine says, "Feed the Dog of Courage!"

DAY 1	DAY 2	DAY 3
4 rounds of box breathing	*4 rounds of box breathing*	*4 rounds of box breathing*
4 rounds of nadi shodhana (alt. nostril breathing)	*4 rounds of nadi shodhana (alt. nostril breathing)*	*4 rounds of nadi shodhana (alt. nostril breathing)*
20 min. of meditation	*20 min. of meditation*	*20 min. of meditation*
Eyes closed: 10 reps of mantra or affirmation	*Eyes closed: 10 reps of mantra or affirmation*	*Eyes closed: 10 reps of mantra or affirmation*
First words	*First words*	*First words*

DAY 1

BASELINE WORKOUT

AMRAP in 10:00 of:

  20 squats

  Toes-to-bar, 10 reps

  20 push-ups

  10 pull-ups

From 10:00 to 15:00:

  Find your 1 rep max clean and jerk

DAY 2

AMRAP MASH-UP TEST #1

AMRAP in 1:00 of double under

Rest 1:00

AMRAP in 1:00 of kettlebell swing (men: 53 lb. / women: 35 lb.)

Rest 2:00 and determine your 40% threshold

EMOM for 14:00 (7 rounds of each):

  Odd min. = 40% threshold for double under

  Even min. = 40% threshold for kettlebell swing

DAY 3

Thruster, 5,3,1,1,1 reps (work up to a 1RM weight)

Rest 2:00 and find your 60% threshold of 1RM

AMRAP in 12:00 of:

  Run 400m (or row 400m)

  10 burpees over barbell (lateral jumps over barbell)

  Thruster, 5 reps (60% 1RM)

TERMINOLOGY

Box breathing = 4-count breathing exercise (see page 176)

Mantra or affirmation = your personal belief statement (see page 181)

First words = the warrior practice of mindful speaking (see page 146)

AMRAP = as many rounds (or reps) as possible

Threshold = your 100% max effort

EMOM = every minute on the minute

RM = 1 rep max effort

DAY 4

4 rounds of box breathing

4 rounds of nadi shodhana (alt. nostril breathing)

20 min. of meditation

Eyes closed: 10 reps of mantra or affirmation

First words

Fitness Outside the Box (walk, run, hike, swim, surf, play!)

Spend 15:00 practicing your overhead squat and Satvana yoga series

DAY 5

4 rounds of box breathing

4 rounds of nadi shodhana (alt. nostril breathing)

20 min. of meditation

Eyes closed: 10 reps of mantra or affirmation

First words

AMRAP MASH-UP TEST #2

AMRAP in 1:00 of wall ball (men: 20 lb., 10 ft. / women: 14 lb., 10 ft.)

Rest 1:00

AMRAP in 1:00 of pull-up

Rest 2:00 and determine your 40% threshold

EMOM for 12:00 (6 rounds of each):

Odd min. = 40% threshold for wall ball

Even min. = 40% threshold for pull-up

DAY 6

4 rounds of box breathing

4 rounds of nadi shodhana (alt. nostril breathing)

20 min. of meditation

Eyes closed: 10 reps of mantra or affirmation

First words

AMRAP MASH-UP TEST #3

AMRAP in 1:00 of toes-to-bar

Rest 1:00

AMRAP in 1:00 of box jumps (men: 24 in. / women: 20 in.)

Rest 1:00

AMRAP in 1:00 of Concept2 row (or double under)

Rest 2:00 and determine your 40% threshold

Every 3 min. for 15:00 (5 rounds each):

Min. 1 = 40% threshold for toes-to-bar

Min. 2 = 40% threshold for box jump

Min. 3 = 40% threshold for Concept2 row

DAY 7

4 rounds of box breathing

4 rounds of nadi shodhana (alt. nostril breathing)

20 min. of meditation

Eyes closed: 10 reps of mantra or affirmation

First words

Bench press, 5,3,1,1,1 reps (work up to 1RM bench press)

Back squat, 5,3,1,1,1 reps (work up to a 1RM squat)

Rest 2:00 and determine 50% of 1RM bench and 1RM squat

4 rounds for time:

Run 400m (or row 400m)

Back squat, 15 reps (50% 1RM)

Bench press, 12 reps (50% 1RM)

2 rope climbs, 15 ft. (or 12 pull-ups)

21-DAY ADVANCED PLAN *(Continued)*

DAY 8	DAY 9	DAY 10	DAY 11
4 rounds of box breathing	*4 rounds of box breathing*	*4 rounds of box breathing*	*4 rounds of box breathing*
4 rounds of nadi shodhana (alt. nostril breathing)	*4 rounds of nadi shodhana (alt. nostril breathing)*	*4 rounds of nadi shodhana (alt. nostril breathing)*	*4 rounds of nadi shodhana (alt. nostril breathing)*
20 min. of meditation	*20 min. of meditation*	*20 min. of meditation*	*20 min. of meditation*
Eyes closed: 10 reps of mantra or affirmation	*Eyes closed: 10 reps of mantra or affirmation*	*Eyes closed: 10 reps of mantra or affirmation*	*Eyes closed: 10 reps of mantra or affirmation*
First words	*First words*	*First words*	*First words*

DAY 8

Fitness Outside the Box (walk, run, hike, swim, surf, play!)

Spend 15:00 on Satvana yoga and practicing your overhead squat

DAY 9

AMRAP MASH-UP EVOLUTION #1 (FORMERLY TEST #1)

EMOM for 14:00 (7 rounds of each):

Odd min. = 50% threshold for double under

Even min. = 50% threshold for kettlebell swing

DAY 10

Clean and jerk, 5,3,1,1,1 reps (work up to a 1RM weight)

Rest 2:00 and find your 60% threshold of 1RM

On a 10:00 running clock:

Clean and jerk, 30 reps (60% 1RM)

Burpee and pull-up, 30 reps

Clean and jerk, AMRAP (60% 1RM)

Note: For this workout, your "score" is your final set of clean and jerks. A "burpee and pull-up" means a full range of motion burpee, then as you jump into the air, instead of clapping your hands, grab the pull-up bar, and complete a pull-up. Come off the bar, and repeat for the prescribed repetitions.

DAY 11

AMRAP MASH-UP EVOLUTION #2 (FORMERLY TEST #2)

EMOM for 12:00 (6 rounds of each):

Odd min. = 50% threshold for wall ball

Even min. = 50% threshold for pull-up

DAY 12

4 rounds of box breathing

4 rounds of nadi shodhana (alt. nostril breathing)

20 min. of meditation

Eyes closed: 10 reps of mantra or affirmation

First words

Fitness Outside the Box (walk, run, hike, swim, surf, play!)

Complete the full Satvana yoga series

DAY 13

4 rounds of box breathing

4 rounds of nadi shodhana (alt. nostril breathing)

20 min. of meditation

Eyes closed: 10 reps of mantra or affirmation

First words

AMRAP MASH-UP EVOLUTION #3 (FORMERLY TEST #3)

Every 3 min. for 15:00 (5 rounds each):

Min. 1 = 50% threshold for toes-to-bar

Min. 2 = 50% threshold for box jump (men: 24 in. / women: 20 in.)

Min. 3 = 50% threshold for Concept2 row

DAY 14

4 rounds of box breathing

4 rounds of nadi shodhana (alt. nostril breathing)

20 min. of meditation

Eyes closed: 10 reps of mantra or affirmation

First words

Shoulder press, 5,3,1,1,1 reps (establish a 1RM)

Rest 2:00 and determine 50% of your 1RM press

4 rounds for time:

Run 400m (or row 400m)

Push press, 15 reps (50% 1RM)

Single-leg squat, 20 reps, 10 each leg

Note: Although the 1RM that you will establish is your press, in the workout, utilize the push press.

DAY 15

4 rounds of box breathing

4 rounds of nadi shodhana (alt. nostril breathing)

20 min. of meditation

Eyes closed: 10 reps of mantra or affirmation

First words

AMRAP MASH-UP EVOLUTION #1 (FORMERLY TEST #1)

EMOM for 12:00 (6 rounds of each):

Odd min. = 60% threshold for double under

Even min. = 60% threshold for kettlebell swing (men: 53 lb. / women: 35 lb.)

DAY 16

4 rounds of box breathing

4 rounds of nadi shodhana (alt. nostril breathing)

20 min. of meditation

Eyes closed: 10 reps of mantra or affirmation

First words

Fitness Outside the Box (walk, run, hike, swim, surf, play!)

Complete the full Satvana yoga series and spend 10:00 practicing your overhead squat

DAY 17

4 rounds of box breathing

4 rounds of nadi shodhana (alt. nostril breathing)

20 min. of meditation

Eyes closed: 10 reps of mantra or affirmation

First words

AMRAP in 20:00 of:

Run 400m (or row 400m)

10 burpees over barbell (lateral jumps over barbell)

Thruster, 5 reps (70% 1RM)

DAY 18

4 rounds of box breathing

4 rounds of nadi shodhana (alt. nostril breathing)

20 min. of meditation

Eyes closed: 10 reps of mantra or affirmation

First words

Deadlift, 5,3,1,1,1 reps (establish a 1RM)

Rest 4:00 and determine 60% 1RM deadlift

For time:

Deadlift, 21 reps (60% 1RM)

Ring dip, 21 reps

Deadlift, 15 reps

Ring dip, 15 reps

Deadlift, 9 reps

Ring dip, 9 reps

DAY 19

4 rounds of box breathing

4 rounds of nadi shodhana (alt. nostril breathing)

20 min. of meditation

Eyes closed: 10 reps of mantra or affirmation

First words

---

1 round for time:

Run 800m

Power clean, 50 reps (50% of 1RM clean and jerk)

30 handstand push-ups

DAY 20

4 rounds of box breathing

4 rounds of nadi shodhana (alt. nostril breathing)

20 min. of meditation

Eyes closed: 10 reps of mantra or affirmation

First words

Fitness Outside the Box (walk, run, hike, swim, surf, play!)

Complete the full Satvana yoga series and spend 10:00 practicing your overhead squat

DAY 21

4 rounds of box breathing

4 rounds of nadi shodhana (alt. nostril breathing)

20 min. of meditation

Eyes closed: 10 reps of mantra or affirmation

First words

BASELINE RETEST

AMRAP in 10:00 of:

    20 squats

    Toes-to-bar, 10 reps

    20 push-ups

    10 pull-ups

From 10:00 to 15:00:

    Find your 1 rep max clean and jerk

Go back to AMRAP Mash-Up Tests 1, 2, and 3, and retest your AMRAP potential. You will be happy to see an improvement in your capacity. Then, repeat the remaining workouts, recalculating your threshold accordingly. You will follow the same protocol for your weight lifting workouts. Every three months, take a week off and just practice yoga, and enjoy Fitness Outside the Box.

AN ONGOING PROGRAM

You've just created an amazing amount of momentum in your life and begun the process of integrating your mind, body, and spirit. Your 21-day challenge can now become a measurable and repeatable fitness plan. Here is how it works:

After finishing 21 days, start over. As you repeat AMRAP Mash-Up Tests 1, 2, and 3, you will be able to measure your performance gains.

You can rotate in and out a variety of movements into the mash-ups and strength components. For a complete list of exercises, along with video demonstrations, go to www.firebreatherfitness.org. You'll also find a series of suggested 21-day cycles for the beginner, intermediate, and advanced athlete.

You will be happy to see an improvement in your capacity. Then, repeat the remaining workouts, recalculating your threshold accordingly. You will follow the same protocol for your weight lifting workouts.

Restoration. Every three months, take a week off and just practice yoga and enjoy Fitness Outside the Box.

Scaled and advanced 21-day cycles. Do you need a 21-day program more within your reach? Or one that's more challenging? Go to www.firebreatherfitness.org for a whiteboard talk on the plan and additional versions that will match your current level.

JOURNALING

I strongly suggest keeping a journal, recording your efforts and impressions from each workout. I've kept mine for 16 years and recorded my very first workout with Coach Glassman in December 2001. Nothing is better than looking back over years of journals and seeing solid proof of improvements made, challenges surpassed, and goals accomplished. It's both useful and rewarding to look back and see how far you've come! In addition to tracking your workout data, I suggest taking a few minutes each morning to write down your daily goals, and to review your purpose, values, and intentions. Then in the evening, mentally review your day and write down three people, accomplishments, experiences, or events you are grateful for. The burning question in your mind should be, "What ELSE am I grateful for?" By continually reflecting on what you are grateful for, a unique thing happens: You attract into your life more things to be grateful for! Contemplate how you can move the direction of your life one degree closer to your purpose. Let this question help focus your goals and intentions for the next day.

STA

NDARDS

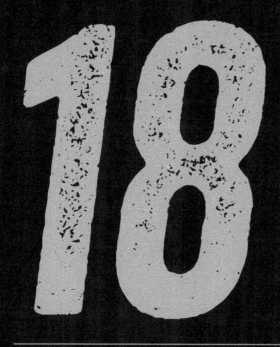

18

FIREBREATHER STANDARDS: TAKING IT TO THE NEXT LEVEL

THE FIREBREATHER FITNESS PROGRAM traces its roots to helping athletes prepare for the demands of combat—mainly, mixed martial arts competitions and "real world" combat such as military and law-enforcement operations. However, it's not just martial artists and professional warrior athletes who can benefit from a progressive ranking system. We all need goals in order to propel us forward.

I believe that having this structure offers both a level of directional guidance as well as defined targets to shoot for. It will also help you stay the course in a comprehensive way and avoid the mistake of focusing on your strengths while letting weaknesses lag behind. Through benchmark workouts and tests across the board—open, close, push, and pull movement categories and conditioning tests—you will see that I have laid out levels of achievement for you to shoot for that correspond with your age and skill level. The Firebreather Fitness ranking system is a tool you can use to ensure many years of challenge, advancement, and accomplishment.

Perhaps most important, it makes a game out of your training. It makes it fun and satisfying as you work your way up the ladder. There's perhaps no better source of motivation for your training than when you ascend a hilltop and can see how far you've come. It's a great confidence-builder. You'll immediately look up at the next level and charge ahead!

The Firebreather Standards in this book are divided into levels (1–3), as well as defined by gender and age. The exercises themselves are sectioned by type—open, close, push, and pull, plus what I define as "conditioning," which refers to a combination of stamina, endurance, speed, and power. Also, note that rather than prescribing a specific weight to utilize on the barbell skills, you are training at a percentage of your relative strength.

Levels 1 and 2 are designed to be achievable within 6 months to 1 year of dedicated training and mindful nutrition. Many who accomplish level 2 will find themselves in the best shape of their lives. I have included levels 1 through 3 here for reference. However, for those Firebreathers who are supercommitted, the upper ranks—levels 4 and 5—await. You can find them at www.firebreatherfitness.org.

You'll notice that there are certain advanced movements that appear in the pages that follow that we didn't cover in the book. In particular, rope climbs and the gymnastics-style muscle-ups (a combination of a ring pull-up and a ring dip) are listed. Muscle-ups are technical movements that can be intimidating at first. But it's a matter of perspective: For the beginner, a single strict pull-up can be intimidating. Perhaps even a single push-up. But that's OK. In fact, it's great. Where body, mind, and spirit truly come together is where you gather up the courage and take on goals and challenges that are outside of your comfort zone. The payoff is that when you crack it open and get that first pull-up, rope climb, or muscle-up, the belief in yourself pours in and opens up all sorts of new possibilities. And this personal belief resonates throughout every corner of your life, both inside and outside the gym.

Also, please note that there are two named workouts, "Helen" and "Karen." These are original, old-school CrossFit workouts created by

Coach Greg Glassman, and I love them! They are comprised of movements you have learned in the book, but combined in a fun, unique way.

For the movements not taught in the Body section of this book, I have a series of videos and how-to information waiting for you on the website www.firebreatherfitness.org. When you're ready to take on these goals, you'll find clear, step-by-step guidance to help you succeed at earning your highest achievement possible. I encourage you to visit the website, where I provide updates and additions to the ranking system on a regular basis. This online community will tie you into the worldwide Firebreather Fitness program and provide you with the inspiration and continued education you need to be at your best.

LEVEL 1: OPEN MEN (18–35)

	BEGINNER	INTERMEDIATE	ADVANCED
OPEN	50 air squats (sub 3:00) ½ body-weight back squat *5 reps* 10 box jumps, 24 in. (sub 1:00) body-weight deadlift *5 reps*	75 air squats (sub 3:00) ¾ body-weight back squat *5 reps* 15 box jumps, 24 in. (sub 1:00) body-weight deadlift *10 reps*	100 air squats (sub 3:00) body-weight back squat *10 reps* 20 box jumps, 24 in. (sub 1:00) body-weight deadlift *21 reps*
CLOSE	knees-to-elbow *10 reps*	knees-to-elbow *15 reps*	knees-to-elbow *21 reps* toes-to-bar *10 reps*
PUSH	25 push-ups, consecutive ½ body-weight bench press *5 reps* ½ body-weight press *1 rep*	35 push-ups, consecutive body-weight bench press *7 reps* ½ body-weight press *5 reps*	50 push-ups, consecutive body-weight bench press *10 reps* ½ body-weight press *10 reps*
PULL	1 pull-up, strict ½ body-weight power clean *1 rep*	3 pull-ups, strict ¾ body-weight power clean *1 rep*	5 pull-ups, strict body-weight power clean *1 rep* 1 rope climb, 15 ft.

CONDITIONING	**"Helen" (sub 20:00)**
	3 rounds for time:
	  400m run
	  kettlebell swing (53 lb.) *21 reps*
	  12 pull-ups
	2-mile run (sub 20:00)
	500m row (sub 2:00)
		"Helen" (sub 18:30)
		3 rounds for time:
		  400m run
		  kettlebell swing (53 lb.) *21 reps*
		  12 pull-ups
		2-mile run (sub 18:30)
		500m row (sub 1:55)
			"Helen" (sub 17:30)
			3 rounds for time:
			  400m run
			  kettlebell swing (53 lb.) *21 reps*
			  12 Pull-Ups
			2-mile run (sub 18:10)
			500m row (sub 1:50)

Note: Unless otherwise stated, all reps are consecutive. Repetition requirements within a specific time frame can be partitioned as necessary.

LEVEL 2: OPEN MEN (18–35)

	BEGINNER	INTERMEDIATE	ADVANCED
OPEN	body-weight back squat *15 reps* 25 box jumps, 24 in. (sub 1:00) 225 lb. deadlift *9 reps*	body-weight back squat *21 reps* 30 box jumps, 24 in. (sub 1:00) 225 lb. deadlift *15 reps*	body-weight back squat *30 reps* 20 box jumps, 30 in. (sub 1:00) 225 lb. deadlift *21 reps*
CLOSE	knees-to-elbow *25 reps* toes-to-bar *15 reps*	toes-to-bar *20 reps*	toes-to-bar *25 reps*
PUSH	50 push-ups, consecutive body-weight bench press *12 reps* 95 lb. press *9 reps*	7 ring dips body-weight bench press *15 reps* 95 lb. press *12 reps*	10 ring dips body-weight bench press *20 reps* 10 handstand push-ups
PULL	7 pull-ups, strict 3 rope climbs, 15 ft. (sub 1:30) body-weight power clean *1 rep*	10 pull-ups, strict 3 rope climbs, 15 ft. (sub 1:15) body-weight power clean *3 reps*	15 pull-ups, strict 3 rope climbs, 15 ft. (sub 1:00) 1 L-sit rope climb, 15 ft. body-weight power clean *5 reps*

CONDITIONING	"Helen" (sub 16:00)
	3 rounds for time:
	  400m run
	  kettlebell swing (53 lb.) *21 reps*
	  12 pull-ups
	2-mile run (sub 14:30)
	500m row (sub 1:45)
		"Helen" (sub 12:00)
		3 rounds for time:
		  400m run
		  kettlebell swing (53 lb.) *21 reps*
		  12 pull-ups
		2-mile run (sub 14:20)
		500m row (sub 1:42)
			"Helen" (sub 10:30)
			3 rounds for time:
			  400m run
			  kettlebell swing (53 lb.) *21 reps*
			  12 pull-ups
			2-mile run (sub 14:10)
			500m row (sub 1:40)
			100 double unders (sub 1:00)

Note: Unless otherwise stated, all reps are consecutive. Repetition requirements within a specific time frame can be partitioned as necessary.

LEVEL 3: OPEN MEN (18–35)

	BEGINNER	INTERMEDIATE	ADVANCED
OPEN	single-leg squat, each leg (sub 1:30) *8 reps* 1½ body-weight back squat *9 reps* 275 lb. deadlift *9 reps* ½ body-weight overhead squat *9 reps*	single-leg squat, each leg (sub 1:30) *12 reps* 1½ body-weight back squat *12 reps* 275 lb. deadlift *12 reps* body-weight overhead squat *7 reps*	single-leg squat, each leg (sub 1:30) *16 reps* 1½ body-weight back squat *15 reps* 275 lb. deadlift *15 reps* body-weight overhead squat *10 reps*
CLOSE	toes-to-bar *30 reps*	toes-to-bar (sub 1:00) *40 reps*	toes-to-bar (sub 1:00) *45 reps*
PUSH	1 muscle-up 1½ body-weight bench press *1 rep* ½ body-weight thruster *15 reps*	3 muscle-ups (sub 1:00) 1½ body-weight bench press *3 reps* ½ body-weight thruster *20 reps*	5 muscle-ups (sub 1:30) 1½ body-weight bench press *5 reps* ½ body-weight thruster *30 reps* 21 handstand push-ups
PULL	20 pull-ups, strict 3 pull-ups, weighted (35 lb.) 1¼ body-weight power clean *1 rep*	10 pull-ups, chest to bar (kipping) 5 pull-ups, weighted (35 lb.) 1½ body-weight power clean (sub 1:30) *2 reps*	15 pull-ups, chest to bar (kipping) 7 pull-ups, weighted (53 lb.) 1½ body-weight power clean (sub 1:30) *3 reps* 2 L-sit rope climbs, 15 ft. (sub 1:00)

CONDITIONING	**"Helen" (sub 10:00)**
	3 rounds for time:
	  400m run
	  kettlebell swing (53 lb.) *21 reps*
	  12 pull-ups
	2-mile run (sub 12:40)
	
	"Karen" (sub 10:00)
	For time:
	  150 wall ball shots (20 lb., 10 ft.)
		"Helen" (sub 9:30)
		3 rounds for time:
		  400m run
		  kettlebell swing (53 lb.) *21 reps*
		  12 pull-ups
		2-mile run (sub 12:35)
		
		"Karen" (sub 8:00)
		For time:
		  150 wall ball shots (20 lb., 10 ft.)
			"Helen" (sub 9:15)
			3 rounds for time:
			  400m run
			  kettlebell swing (53 lb.) *21 reps*
			  12 pull-ups
			2-mile run (sub 12:30)
			
			"Karen" (sub 7:00)
			For time:
			  150 wall ball shots (20 lb., 10 ft.)

Note: Unless otherwise stated, all reps are consecutive. Repetition requirements within a specific time frame can be partitioned as necessary.

LEVEL 1: MASTERS MEN (36–45)

	BEGINNER	INTERMEDIATE	ADVANCED
OPEN	50 air squats (sub 3:00) ½ body-weight back squat *5 reps* 10 box jumps, 24 in. (sub 1:00) body-weight deadlift *5 reps*	75 air squats (sub 3:00) ¾ body-weight back squat *5 reps* 15 box jumps, 24 in. (sub 1:00) body-weight deadlift *10 reps*	100 air squats (sub 3:00) body-weight back squat *10 reps* 20 box jumps, 24 in. (sub 1:00) body-weight deadlift *15 reps*
CLOSE	knees-to-elbow *10 reps*	knees-to-elbow *15 reps*	knees-to-elbow *21 reps* toes-to-bar *10 reps*
PUSH	25 push-ups, consecutive body-weight bench press *5 reps* ½ body-weight press *1 rep*	35 push-ups, consecutive body-weight bench press *7 reps* ½ body-weight press *5 reps*	50 push-ups, consecutive body-weight bench press *10 reps* ½ body-weight press *10 reps*
PULL	1 pull-up, strict ½ body-weight power clean *1 rep*	3 pull-ups, strict ¾ body-weight power clean *1 rep*	5 pull-ups, strict body-weight power clean *1 rep*

CONDITIONING	**"Helen" (sub 20:00)**
	3 rounds for time:
	  400m run
	  kettlebell swing (53 lb.) *21 reps*
	  12 pull-Ups
	2-mile run (sub 20:00)
	500m row (sub 2:00)
		"Helen" (sub 19:00)
		3 rounds for time:
		  400m run
		  kettlebell swing (53 lb.) *21 reps*
		  12 pull-Ups
		2-mile run (sub 19:00)
		500m row (sub 1:57)
			"Helen" (sub 18:00)
			3 rounds for time:
			  400m run
			  kettlebell swing (53 lb.) *21 reps*
			  12 pull-Ups
			2-mile run (sub 18:30)
			500m row (sub 1:55)

Note: Unless otherwise stated, all reps are consecutive. Repetition requirements within a specific time frame can be partitioned as necessary.

LEVEL 2: MASTERS MEN (36–45)

	BEGINNER	INTERMEDIATE	ADVANCED
OPEN	body-weight back squat *15 reps* 25 box jumps, 24 in. (sub 1:00) 225 lb. deadlift *9 reps*	body-weight back squat *21 reps* 30 box jumps, 24 in. (sub 1:00) 225 lb. deadlift *12 reps*	body-weight back squat *25 reps* 20 box jumps, 30 in. (sub 1:00) 225 lb. deadlift *15 reps*
CLOSE	knees-to-elbow *25 reps* toes-to-bar *15 reps*	toes-to-bar *20 reps*	toes-to-bar *25 reps*
PUSH	5 ring dips body-weight bench press *10 reps* 95 lb. press *9 reps*	7 ring dips body-weight bench press *12 reps* 95 lb. press *11 reps*	10 ring dips body-weight bench press *15 reps* 10 handstand push-ups
PULL	12 pull-ups, strict 3 rope climbs, 15 ft. (sub 1:30) body-weight power clean *1 rep*	15 pull-ups, strict 3 rope climbs, 15 ft. (sub 1:15) body-weight power clean *3 reps*	20 pull-ups, strict 3 rope climbs, 15 ft. (sub 1:00) 1 L-sit rope climb, 15 ft. body-weight power clean *5 reps*
CONDITIONING	**"Helen" (sub 16:00)** 3 rounds for time: 400m run kettlebell swing (53 lb.) *21 reps* 12 pull-ups 2-mile run (sub 15:00) 500m row (sub 1:45)	**"Helen" (sub 13:00)** 3 rounds for time: 400m run kettlebell swing (53 lb.) *21 reps* 12 pull-ups 2-mile run (sub 14:30) 500m row (sub 1:42)	**"Helen" (sub 11:00)** 3 rounds for time: 400m run kettlebell swing (53 lb.) *21 reps* 12 pull-ups 2-mile run (sub 14:20) 500m row (sub 1:40) 100 double unders (sub 1:00)

Note: Unless otherwise stated, all reps are consecutive. Repetition requirements within a specific time frame can be partitioned as necessary.

LEVEL 3: MASTERS MEN (36–45)

	BEGINNER	INTERMEDIATE	ADVANCED
OPEN	single-leg squat, each leg (sub 1:30) *8 reps* 1½ body-weight back squat *9 reps* 275 lb. deadlift *6 reps* ½ body-weight overhead squat *9 reps*	single-leg squat, each leg (sub 1:30) *12 reps* 1½ body-weight back squat *12 reps* 275 lb. deadlift *10 reps* ½ body-weight overhead squat *15 reps*	single-leg squat, each leg (sub 1:30) *16 reps* 1½ body-weight back squat *15 reps* 275 lb. deadlift *12 reps* body-weight overhead squat *12 reps*
CLOSE	toes-to-bar *30 reps*	toes-to-bar (sub 1:00) *35 reps*	toes-to-bar (sub 1:00) *40 reps*
PUSH	1 muscle-up 1½ body-weight bench press *1 rep* ½ body-weight thruster *12 reps*	3 muscle-ups (sub 1:00) 1½ body-weight bench press *3 reps* ½ body-weight thruster *15 reps*	5 muscle-ups (sub 1:30) 1½ body-weight bench press *5 reps* ½ body-weight thruster *25 reps* 12 handstand push-ups
PULL	20 pull-ups, strict 3 pull-ups, weighted (35 lb.) 1¼ body-weight power clean *1 rep*	10 pull-ups, chest to bar (kipping) 5 pull-ups, weighted (35 lb.) 1¼ body-weight power clean (sub 1:30) *2 reps*	15 pull-ups, chest to bar (kipping) 3 pull-ups, weighted (53 lb.) 1¼ body-weight power clean (sub 1:30) *3 reps* 1 L-sit rope climb, 15 ft.

CONDITIONING	**"Helen" (sub 10:45)**
	3 rounds for time:
	  400m run
	  kettlebell swing (53 lb.) *21 reps*
	  12 pull-ups
	2-mile run (sub 14:00)
	
	"Karen" (sub 10:00)
	For time:
	  150 wall ball shots (20 lb., 10 ft.)
		"Helen" (sub 10:00)
		3 rounds for time:
		  400m run
		  kettlebell swing (53 lb.) *21 reps*
		  12 pull-ups
		2-mile run (sub 13:30)
		
		"Karen" (sub 8:30)
		For time:
		  150 wall ball shots (20 lb., 10 ft.)
			"Helen" (sub 9:30)
			3 rounds for time:
			  400m run
			  kettlebell swing (53 lb.) *21 reps*
			  12 pull-ups
			2-mile run (sub 13:00)
			
			"Karen" (sub 7:30)
			For time:
			  150 wall ball shots (20 lb., 10 ft.)

Note: Unless otherwise stated, all reps are consecutive. Repetition requirements within a specific time frame can be partitioned as necessary.

LEVEL 1: MASTERS 2 MEN (46–54)

	BEGINNER	INTERMEDIATE	ADVANCED
OPEN	30 air squats (sub 3:00) ½ body-weight back squat *5 reps* 10 box jumps/steps, 24 in. (sub 1:00) body-weight deadlift *1 rep*	50 air squats (sub 3:00) ½ body-weight back squat *5 reps* 15 box jumps/steps, 24 in. (sub 1:00) body-weight deadlift *5 reps*	75 air squats (sub 3:00) ½ body-weight back squat *10 reps* 20 box jumps/steps, 24 in. (sub 1:00) body-weight deadlift *9 reps*
CLOSE	knees-to-elbow *5 reps*	knees-to-elbow *7 reps*	knees-to-elbow *10 reps*
PUSH	10 push-ups, consecutive ½ body-weight bench press *5 reps* ½ body-weight press *1 rep*	20 push-ups, consecutive ½ body-weight bench press *9 reps* ½ body-weight press *3 reps*	30 push-ups, consecutive body-weight bench press *12 reps* ½ body-weight press *5 reps*
PULL	1 pull-up, strict 1 rope climb, 15 ft. ½ body-weight power clean *1 rep*	3 pull-ups, strict 1 rope climb, 15 ft. ¾ body-weight power clean *1 rep*	5 pull-ups, strict 2 rope climbs, 15 ft. (sub 1:30) body-weight power clean *1 rep*

CONDITIONING	**"Helen" (sub 25:00)**
	3 rounds for time:
	  400m run
	  kettlebell swing (53 lb.) *21 reps*
	  12 pull-ups
	2-mile run (sub 20:00)
	500m row (sub 2:30)
		"Helen" (sub 23:00)
		3 rounds for time:
		  400m run
		  kettlebell swing (53 lb.) *21 reps*
		  12 pull-ups
		2-mile run (sub 19:30)
		500m row (sub 2:20)
			"Helen" (sub 22:00)
			3 rounds for time:
			  400m run
			  kettlebell swing (53 lb.) *21 reps*
			  12 pull-ups
			2-mile run (sub 19:00)
			500m row (sub 2:10)

Note: Unless otherwise stated, all reps are consecutive. Repetition requirements within a specific time frame can be partitioned as necessary.

LEVEL 2: MASTERS 2 MEN (46–54)

	BEGINNER	INTERMEDIATE	ADVANCED
OPEN	body-weight back squat *9 reps* 21 box steps, 24 in. (sub 1:00) body-weight deadlift *10 reps*	body-weight back squat *12 reps* 23 box steps, 24 in. (sub 1:00) body-weight deadlift *12 reps*	body-weight back squat *15 reps* 25 box steps, 24 in. (sub 1:00) body-weight deadlift *15 reps*
CLOSE	knees-to-elbow *11 reps* toes-to-bar *5 reps*	knees-to-elbow *12 reps* toes-to-bar *7 reps*	knees-to-elbow *15 reps* toes-to-bar *10 reps*
PUSH	35 push-ups, consecutive body-weight bench press *7 reps* 95 lb. press *5 reps*	40 push-ups, consecutive body-weight bench press *9 reps* 95 lb. press *7 reps*	45 push-ups, consecutive body-weight bench press *10 reps* 95 lb. press *9 reps*
PULL	11 pull-ups, strict 3 rope climbs, 15 ft. (sub 1:30) body-weight power clean (sub 1:30) *2 reps*	12 pull-ups, strict 3 rope climbs, 15 ft. (sub 1:30) body-weight power clean (sub 1:30) *3 reps*	13 pull-ups, strict 3 rope climbs, 15 ft. (sub 1:30) body-weight power clean (sub 1:30) *5 reps*

CONDITIONING	**"Helen" (sub 20:00)**
	3 rounds for time:
	  400m run
	  kettlebell swing (53 lb.) *21 reps*
	  12 pull-ups
	2-mile run (sub 18:30)
	500m row (sub 2:30)
		"Helen" (sub 19:00)
		3 rounds for time:
		  400m run
		  kettlebell swing (53 lb.) *21 reps*
		  12 pull-ups
		2-mile run (sub 18:00)
		500m row (sub 2:10)
			"Helen" (sub 18:00)
			3 rounds for time:
			  400m run
			  kettlebell swing (53 lb.) *21 reps*
			  12 pull-ups
			2-mile run (sub 17:30)
			500m row (sub 1:55)

Note: Unless otherwise stated, all reps are consecutive. Repetition requirements within a specific time frame can be partitioned as necessary.

LEVEL 3: MASTERS 2 MEN (46–54)

	BEGINNER	INTERMEDIATE	ADVANCED
OPEN	body-weight back squat *15 reps* body-weight deadlift *21 reps* 25 box steps, 24 in. (sub 1:00)	½ body-weight overhead squat *9 reps* 1½ body-weight deadlift *10 reps* 15 box steps, 30 in. (sub 1:30)	½ body-weight overhead squat *12 reps* 1½ body-weight deadlift *12 reps* 21 box steps, 30 in. (sub 1:30)
CLOSE	knees-to-elbow *20 reps* toes-to-bar *15 reps*	toes-to-bar *20 reps*	toes-to-bar *25 reps*
PUSH	45 push-ups body-weight bench press *15 reps* 95 lb. press *9 reps*	50 push-ups 1 handstand hold (1:00) 1¼ body-weight bench press *3 reps*	1 muscle-up 5 handstand push-ups 1½ body-weight bench press *1 rep*
PULL	12 pull-ups, strict 3 rope climbs, 15 ft. (sub 1:30) body-weight power clean (sub 1:30) *5 reps*	10 pull-ups, chest to bar (kipping) 3 rope climbs, 15 ft. (sub 1:00) body-weight power clean (sub 2:00) *7 reps*	15 pull-ups, chest to bar (kipping) 1 L-sit rope climb, 15 ft. body-weight power clean (sub 2:00) *9 reps*

CONDITIONING	**"Helen" (sub 17:30)**
	3 rounds for time:
	  400m run
	  kettlebell swing (53 lb.) *21 reps*
	  12 pull-ups
	2-mile run (sub 17:00)
	500m row (sub 1:50)
		"Helen" (sub 17:00)
		3 rounds for time:
		  400m run
		  kettlebell swing (53 lb.) *21 reps*
		  12 pull-ups
		2-mile run (sub 16:00)
		500m row (sub 1:45)
			"Helen" (sub 15:00)
			3 rounds for time:
			  400m run
			  kettlebell swing (53 lb.) *21 reps*
			  12 pull-ups
			2-mile run (sub 14:00)
			"Karen" (sub 14:00)
			For time:
			  150 wall ball shots (20 lb., 10 ft.)

Note: Unless otherwise stated, all reps are consecutive. Repetition requirements within a specific time frame can be partitioned as necessary.

LEVEL 1: OPEN WOMEN (18—35)

	BEGINNER	INTERMEDIATE	ADVANCED
OPEN	50 air squats (sub 3:00) ½ body-weight back squat *5 reps* 10 box jumps, 20 in. (sub 1:00) body-weight deadlift *5 reps*	75 air squats (sub 3:00) ¾ body-weight back squat *5 reps* 15 box jumps, 20 in. (sub 1:00) body-weight deadlift *7 reps*	100 air squats (sub 3:00) body-weight back squat *10 reps* 20 box jumps, 20 in. (sub 1:00) body-weight deadlift *9 reps*
CLOSE	knees-to-elbow *10 reps*	knees-to-elbow *15 reps*	knees-to-elbow *21 reps* toes-to-bar *10 reps*
PUSH	10 push-ups ¼ body-weight bench press *3 reps* ¼ body-weight press *1 rep*	15 push-ups ¼ body-weight bench press *5 reps* ¼ body-weight press *5 reps*	20 push-ups ¼ body-weight bench press *7 reps* ½ body-weight press *10 reps*
PULL	10 ring rows 1 rope climb, 15 ft. ¼ body-weight power clean *1 rep*	20 ring rows 1 rope climb, 15 ft. ½ body-weight power clean *1 rep*	1 pull-up, strict 2 rope climbs, 15 ft. (sub 2:00) body-weight power clean *1 rep*

CONDITIONING	**"Helen" (sub 20:00)**
	3 rounds for time:
	  400m run
	  kettlebell swing (35 lb.) *21 reps*
	  12 pull-ups
	2-mile run (sub 20:00)
	500m row (sub 2:30)
		"Helen" (sub 18:30)
		3 rounds for time:
		  400m run
		  kettlebell swing (35 lb.) *21 reps*
		  12 pull-ups
		2-mile run (sub 19:00)
		500m row (sub 2:20)
			"Helen" (sub 18:00)
			3 rounds for time:
			  400m run
			  kettlebell swing (35 lb.) *21 reps*
			  12 pull-ups
			2-mile run (sub 18:30)
			500m row (sub 2:10)

Note: Unless otherwise stated, all reps are consecutive. Repetition requirements within a specific time frame can be partitioned as necessary.

LEVEL 2: OPEN WOMEN (18–35)

	BEGINNER	INTERMEDIATE	ADVANCED
OPEN	body-weight back squat *15 reps* 25 box jumps, 20 in. (sub 1:00) 165 lb. deadlift (sub 3:00) *9 reps*	body-weight back squat *18 reps* 30 box jumps, 20 in. (sub 1:00) 165 lb. deadlift (sub 3:00) *15 reps*	body-weight back squat *20 reps* 20 box jumps, 24 in. (sub 1:00) 165 lb. deadlift (sub 3:00) *21 reps*
CLOSE	knees-to-elbow (sub 1:00) *25 reps* toes-to-bar (sub 1:00) *15 reps*	toes-to-bar (sub 1:00) *18 reps*	toes-to-bar (sub 1:00) *20 reps*
PUSH	25 push-ups, consecutive ½ body-weight bench press *9 reps* 3 handstand push-ups, consecutive	30 push-ups, consecutive ½ body-weight bench press *10 reps* 3 handstand push-ups, consecutive	5 ring dips ½ body-weight bench press *12 reps* 5 handstand push-ups (sub 1:00)
PULL	5 pull-ups, strict 2 rope climbs, 15 ft. (sub 1:30) body-weight power clean *1 rep*	7 pull-ups (kipping) 3 rope climbs, 15 ft. (sub 1:15) body-weight power clean *3 reps*	9 pull-ups (kipping) 2 rope climbs, 15 ft. (sub 1:00) body-weight power clean (sub 1:00) *5 reps*

CONDITIONING	**"Helen" (sub 17:00)**
	3 rounds for time:
	  400m run
	  kettlebell swing (35 lb.) *21 reps*
	  12 pull-ups
	2-mile run (sub 16:00)
	500m row (sub 2:00)
		"Helen" (sub 16:00)
		3 rounds for time:
		  400m run
		  kettlebell swing (35 lb.) *21 reps*
		  12 pull-ups
		2-mile run (sub 15:45)
		500m row (sub 1:55)
			"Helen" (sub 14:00)
			3 rounds for time:
			  400m run
			  kettlebell swing (35 lb.) *21 reps*
			  12 pull-ups
			2-mile run (sub 15:00)
			500m row (sub 1:50)

Note: Unless otherwise stated, all reps are consecutive. Repetition requirements within a specific time frame can be partitioned as necessary.

LEVEL 3: OPEN WOMEN (18–35)

	BEGINNER	INTERMEDIATE	ADVANCED
OPEN	single-leg squat, each leg (sub 1:30) *8 reps* 1¼ body-weight back squat *9 reps* 185 lb. deadlift (sub 1:00) *9 reps* ½ body-weight overhead squat *9 reps*	single-leg squat, each leg (sub 1:30) *12 reps* 1¼ body-weight back squat *12 reps* 185 lb. deadlift (sub 1:00) *12 reps* body-weight overhead squat *7 reps*	single-leg squat, each leg (sub 1:30) *16 reps* 1¼ body-weight back squat *15 reps* 185 lb. deadlift (sub 1:00) *15 reps* body-weight overhead squat *10 reps*
CLOSE	toes-to-bar *15 reps*	toes-to-bar *21 reps*	toes-to-bar (sub 1:00) *30 reps*
PUSH	1 muscle-up 1¼ body-weight bench press *1 rep* ½ body-weight thruster *12 reps*	3 muscle-ups (sub 1:00) 1¼ body-weight bench press *3 reps* ½ body-weight thruster *15 reps*	5 muscle-ups (sub 1:30) body-weight bench press *2 reps* ½ body-weight thruster *21 reps*
PULL	10 pull-ups, strict 3 pull-ups, weighted (25 lb.) 1¼ body-weight power clean *1 rep*	10 pull-ups, chest to bar (kipping) 4 pull-ups, weighted (25 lb.)	15 pull-ups, chest to bar (kipping) 3 pull-ups, weighted (35 lb.) 1¼ body-weight power clean (sub 1:30) *3 reps*

CONDITIONING	**"Helen" (sub 10:25)**
	3 rounds for time:
	  400m run
	  kettlebell swing (35 lb.) *21 reps*
	  12 pull-ups
	2-mile run (sub 14:55)
	500m row (sub 1:50)
		"Helen" (sub 10:15)
		3 rounds for time:
		  400m run
		  kettlebell swing (35 lb.) *21 reps*
		  12 pull-ups
		2-mile run (sub 14:40)
		
		"Karen" (sub 8:00)
		For time:
		  150 wall ball shots (14 lb., 8 ft.)
			"Helen" (sub 10:05)
			3 rounds for time:
			  400m run
			  kettlebell swing (35 lb.) *21 reps*
			  12 pull-ups
			2-mile run (sub 14:30)
			
			"Karen" (sub 8:00)
			For time:
			  150 wall ball shots (14 lb., 8 ft.)

Note: Unless otherwise stated, all reps are consecutive. Repetition requirements within a specific time frame can be partitioned as necessary.

LEVEL 1: MASTERS WOMEN (36–45)

	BEGINNER	INTERMEDIATE	ADVANCED
OPEN	50 air squats (sub 3:00) ½ body-weight back squat *3 reps* 10 box jumps, 20 in. (sub 1:00) body-weight deadlift (sub 3:00) *5 reps*	70 air squats (sub 3:00) ¾ body-weight back squat *4 reps* 15 box jumps, 20 in. (sub 1:00) body-weight deadlift (sub 3:00) *6 reps*	90 air squats (sub 3:00) body-weight back squat *7 reps* 20 box jumps, 20 in. (sub 1:00) body-weight deadlift (sub 3:00) *7 reps*
CLOSE	knees-to-elbow *10 reps*	knees-to-elbow *12 reps*	knees-to-elbow *15 reps* toes-to-bar *5 reps*
PUSH	10 push-ups ¼ body-weight bench press *3 reps* ¼ body-weight press *1 rep*	12 push-ups ¼ body-weight bench press *5 reps* ¼ body-weight press *5 reps*	15 push-ups ¼ body-weight bench press *7 reps* ½ body-weight press *10 reps*
PULL	10 ring rows 1 rope climb, 15 ft. ¼ body-weight power clean *1 rep*	20 ring rows 1 rope climb, 15 ft. ½ body-weight power clean *1 rep*	1 pull-up, strict 1 rope climb, 15 ft. ¾ body-weight power clean *1 rep*

CONDITIONING	**Helen" (sub 20:00)**
	3 rounds for time:
	  400m run
	  kettlebell swing (35 lb.) *21 reps*
	  12 pull-ups
	2-mile run (sub 22:00)
	500m row (sub 2:30)
		"Helen" (sub 19:00)
		3 rounds for time:
		  400m run
		  kettlebell swing (35 lb.) *21 reps*
		  12 pull-ups
		2-mile run (sub 21:00)
		500m row (sub 2:20)
			"Helen" (sub 18:30)
			3 rounds for time:
			  400m run
			  kettlebell swing (35 lb.) *21 reps*
			  12 pull-ups
			2-mile run (sub 20:00)
			500m row (sub 2:10)

Note: Unless otherwise stated, all reps are consecutive. Repetition requirements within a specific time frame can be partitioned as necessary.

LEVEL 2: MASTERS WOMEN (36–45)

	BEGINNER	INTERMEDIATE	ADVANCED
OPEN	body-weight back squat *10 reps* 25 box jumps, 20 in. (sub 1:00) 155 lb. deadlift *9 reps*	body-weight back squat *15 reps* 30 box jumps, 20 in. (sub 1:00) 155 lb. deadlift (sub 3:00) *15 reps*	body-weight back squat *17 reps* 20 box jumps, 24 in. (sub 1:30) 155 lb. deadlift (sub 3:00) *21 reps*
CLOSE	knees-to-elbow *20 reps* toes-to-bar *10 reps*	toes-to-bar (sub 1:00) *15 reps*	toes-to-bar (sub 1:00) *20 reps*
PUSH	17 push-ups ½ body-weight bench press *9 reps* 3 handstand push-ups	7 ring push-ups ½ body-weight bench press *9 reps* 4 handstand push-ups (sub 1:00)	5 ring dips body-weight bench press *1 rep* 5 handstand push-ups (sub 1:00)
PULL	4 pull-ups, strict 2 rope climbs, 15 ft. (sub 1:30) body-weight power clean *1 rep*	5 pull-ups, strict 2 rope climbs, 15 ft. (sub 1:15) body-weight power clean *2 reps*	7 pull-ups, strict 2 rope climbs, 15 ft. (sub 1:00) body-weight power clean (sub 1:00) *3 reps*
CONDITIONING	**"Helen" (sub 16:45)** 3 rounds for time: 400m run kettlebell swing (35 lb.) *21 reps* 12 pull-ups 2-mile run (sub 19:00) 500m row (sub 2:00)	**"Helen" (sub 16:10)** 3 rounds for time: 400m run kettlebell swing (35 lb.) *21 reps* 12 pull-ups 2-mile run (sub 17:00) 500m row (sub 1:55)	**"Helen" (sub 14:30)** 3 rounds for time: 400m run kettlebell swing (35 lb.) *21 reps* 12 pull-ups 2-mile run (sub 16:00) 500m row (sub 1:50)

Note: Unless otherwise stated, all reps are consecutive. Repetition requirements within a specific time frame can be partitioned as necessary.

LEVEL 3: MASTERS WOMEN (36–45)

	BEGINNER	INTERMEDIATE	ADVANCED
OPEN	single-leg squat, each leg (sub 1:30) *6 reps* 1¼ body-weight back squat *9 reps* 175 lb. deadlift *9 reps* ½ body-weight overhead squat *9 reps*	single-leg squat, each leg (sub 1:30) *10 reps* 1¼ body-weight back squat *10 reps* 175 lb. deadlift (sub 1:00) *12 reps* ½ body-weight overhead squat *12 reps*	single-leg squat, each leg (sub 1:30) *14 reps* 1¼ body-weight back squat *12 reps* 175 lb. deadlift (sub 1:00) *15 reps* body-weight overhead squat *7 reps*
CLOSE	toes-to-bar (sub 1:00) *15 reps*	toes-to-bar (sub 1:00) *21 reps*	toes-to-bar (sub 1:00) *30 reps*
PUSH	1 muscle-up 1¼ body-weight bench press *1 rep* ½ body-weight thruster *12 reps*	3 muscle-ups (sub 1:00) ¾ body-weight bench press *3 reps* ½ body-weight thruster *15 reps*	5 muscle-ups (sub 1:30) body-weight bench press *2 reps* ½ body-weight thruster *21 reps*
PULL	9 pull-ups, strict 1 pull-up, weighted (10 lb.) 1¼ body-weight power clean *1 rep*	7 pull-ups, chest to bar (kipping) 2 pull-ups, weighted (25 lb.) 1¼ body-weight power clean (sub 1:30) *2 reps*	10 pull-ups, chest to bar (kipping) 3 pull-ups, weighted (35 lb.) 1¼ body-weight power clean (sub 1:30) *3 reps*
CONDITIONING	**"Helen" (sub 14:00)** 3 rounds for time: 400m run kettlebell swing (35 lb.) *21 reps* 12 pull-ups 2-mile run (sub 15:30) 500m row (sub 1:50)	**"Helen" (sub 13:30)** 3 rounds for time: 400m run kettlebell swing (35 lb.) *21 reps* 12 pull-ups 2-mile run (sub 15:00) **"Karen" (sub 10:15)** For time: 150 wall ball shots (14 lb., 8 ft.)	**"Helen" (sub 12:00)** 3 rounds for time: 400m run kettlebell swing (35 lb.) *21 reps* 12 pull-ups 2-mile run (sub 14:45) **"Karen" (sub 8:00)** For time: 150 wall ball shots (14 lb., 8 ft.)

Note: Unless otherwise stated, all reps are consecutive. Repetition requirements within a specific time frame can be partitioned as necessary.

LEVEL 1: MASTERS 2 WOMEN (46–54)

	BEGINNER	INTERMEDIATE	ADVANCED
OPEN	30 air squats (sub 1:30) ½ body-weight back squat *2 reps* 10 box steps, 20 in. (sub 1:00) body-weight deadlift (sub 3:00) *2 reps*	40 air squats (sub 1:30) ½ body-weight back squat *3 reps* 14 box steps, 20 in. (sub 1:00) body-weight deadlift (sub 3:00) *3 reps*	50 air squats (sub 1:30) ½ body-weight back squat *5 reps* 20 box steps, 20 in. (sub 1:00) body-weight deadlift (sub 3:00) *5 reps*
CLOSE	knees-to-elbow *5 reps*	knees-to-elbow *7 reps*	knees-to-elbow *10 reps*
PUSH	5 push-ups ¼ body-weight bench press *2 reps* ¼ body-weight press *1 rep*	7 push-ups ¼ body-weight bench press *3 reps* ¼ body-weight press *2 reps*	12 push-ups ¼ body-weight bench press *5 reps* ½ body-weight press *3 reps*
PULL	10 ring rows 1 rope climb, 15 ft. ¼ body-weight power clean *1 rep*	15 ring rows 1 rope climb, 15 ft. (sub 2:00) ½ body-weight power clean *2 reps*	20 ring rows 2 rope climbs, 15 ft. (sub 2:00) ¾ body-weight power clean *3 reps*

CONDITIONING	**"Helen" (sub 22:00)**
	3 rounds for time:
	  400m run
	  kettlebell swing (35 lb.) *21 reps*
	  12 pull-ups
	2-mile run (sub 22:00)
	500m row (sub 2:30)
		"Helen" (sub 19:00)
		3 rounds for time:
		  400m run
		  kettlebell swing (35 lb.) *21 reps*
		  12 pull-ups
		2-mile run (sub 21:30)
		500m row (sub 2:20)
			"Helen" (sub 18:30)
			3 rounds for time:
			  400m run
			  kettlebell swing (35 lb.) *21 reps*
			  12 pull-ups
			2-mile run (sub 21:00)
			500m row (sub 2:10)

Note: Unless otherwise stated, all reps are consecutive. Repetition requirements within a specific time frame can be partitioned as necessary.

LEVEL 2: MASTERS 2 WOMEN (46–54)

	BEGINNER	INTERMEDIATE	ADVANCED
OPEN	body-weight back squat *7 reps* 15 box steps, 20 in. (sub 1:00) 155 lb. deadlift (sub 1:00) *9 reps*	body-weight back squat *10 reps* 20 box steps, 20 in. (sub 1:00) 155 lb. deadlift (sub 1:00) *12 reps*	body-weight back squat *12 reps* 25 box steps, 20 in. (sub 1:00) 155 lb. deadlift (sub 1:30) *15 reps*
CLOSE	knees-to-elbow *15 reps* toes-to-bar (sub 1:00) *10 reps*	toes-to-bar (sub 1:00) *10 reps*	toes-to-bar (sub 1:00) *12 reps*
PUSH	15 push-ups ½ body-weight bench press *9 reps* 3 handstand push-ups (sub 1:00)	3 ring push-ups ½ body-weight bench press *12 reps* 5 handstand push-ups (sub 1:00)	3 ring dips ½ body-weight bench press *15 reps* 1 handstand hold (1:00)
PULL	3 pull-ups, strict 2 rope climbs, 15 ft. (sub 1:30) body-weight power clean *1 rep*	4 pull-ups, strict 2 rope climbs, 15 ft. (sub 1:15) body-weight power clean (sub 1:00) *2 reps*	5 pull-ups, strict 2 rope climbs, 15 ft. (sub 1:00) body-weight power clean (sub 1:00) *3 reps*
CONDITIONING	**"Helen" (sub 18:00)** 3 rounds for time: 400m run kettlebell swing (35 lb.) *21 reps* 12 pull-ups 2-mile run (sub 19:30) 500m row (sub 2:05)	**"Helen" (sub 17:00)** 3 rounds for time: 400m run kettlebell swing (35 lb.) *21 reps* 12 pull-ups 2-mile run (sub 19:15) 500m row (sub 2:00)	**"Helen" (sub 15:00)** 3 rounds for time: 400m run kettlebell swing (35 lb.) *21 reps* 12 pull-ups 2-mile run (sub 18:30) 500m row (sub 1:57)

Note: Unless otherwise stated, all reps are consecutive. Repetition requirements within a specific time frame can be partitioned as necessary.

LEVEL 3: MASTERS 2 WOMEN (46–54)

	BEGINNER	INTERMEDIATE	ADVANCED
OPEN	single-leg squat, each leg (sub 1:30) *4 reps* body-weight back squat *9 reps* 155 lb. deadlift *9 reps* ½ body-weight overhead squat *6 reps*	single-leg squat, each leg (sub 1:30) *6 reps* body-weight back squat *12 reps* 155 lb. deadlift (sub 1:00) *12 reps* ½ body-weight overhead squat *9 reps*	single-leg squat, each leg (sub 1:30) *8 reps* body-weight back squat *15 reps* 155 lb. deadlift (sub 1:00) *15 reps* ½ body-weight overhead squat *12 reps*
CLOSE	toes-to-bar *12 reps*	toes-to-bar *15 reps*	toes-to-bar *21 reps*
PUSH	5 pull-ups / 5 ring dips (sub 0:30) body-weight bench press *1 rep* ½ body-weight thruster *10 reps*	7 pull-ups / 7 ring dips (sub 0:30) ¾ body-weight bench press *1 rep* ½ body-weight thruster *15 reps*	1 muscle-up ¾ body-weight bench press *3 reps* ½ body-weight thrusters *21 reps*
PULL	5 pull-ups, strict 1 pull-up, weighted (10 lb.) 1¼ body-weight power clean *1 rep*	7 pull-ups, chest to bar (kipping) 2 pull-ups, weighted (10 lb.) 1¼ body-weight power clean (sub 1:30) *2 reps*	10 pull-ups, chest to bar (kipping) 3 pull-ups, weighted (10 lb.) 1¼ body-weight power clean (sub 1:30) *3 reps*
CONDITIONING	**"Helen" (sub 14:30)** 3 rounds for time: 400m run kettlebell swing (35 lb.) *21 reps* 12 pull-ups 2-mile run (sub 13:45) 500m row (sub 1:55)	**"Helen" (sub 14:00)** 3 rounds for time: 400m run kettlebell swing (35 lb.) *21 reps* 12 pull-ups 2-mile run (sub 13:30) **"Karen" (sub 12:30)** For time: 150 wall ball shots (14 lb., 8 ft.)	**"Helen" (sub 13:00)** 3 rounds for time: 400m run kettlebell swing (35 lb.) *21 reps* 12 pull-ups 2-mile run (sub 13:00) **"Karen" (sub 12:00)** For time: 150 wall ball shots (14 lb., 8 ft.)

Note: Unless otherwise stated, all reps are consecutive. Repetition requirements within a specific time frame can be partitioned as necessary.

Recommended Reading

My goal in writing this book was to provide easy-to-follow lessons and clear steps to enhance life experience and strengthen mind, body, and spirit. If you are interested in deepening your knowledge of self-mastery, goal-setting, and personal success, I recommend the following resources.

Books

Amundson, Greg. *God in Me*. Robertson Publishing, 2016.

Capps, Charles. *The Tongue: A Creative Force*. Tulsa, OK: Harrison House, Inc., 1976.

Carnegie, Dale. *How to Win Friends & Influence People*. New York: Simon & Schuster, 1981.

Divine, Mark. *Kokoro Yoga: Maximize Your Human Potential and Develop the Spirit of a Warrior*. New York: St. Martin's Press, 2016.

—. *Unbeatable Mind: Forge Resiliency and Mental Toughness to Succeed at an Elite Level*. CreateSpace Independent Publishing, 2015.

—. *The Way of the SEAL: Think Like an Elite Warrior to Lead and Succeed*. White Plains, NY: The Reader's Digest Association, Inc., 2013.

Frankl, Viktor E. *Man's Search for Meaning*. Boston: Beacon Press, 1992.

Gates, Rolf. *Meditations from the Mat: Daily Reflections on the Path of Yoga*. New York: Anchor Books, 2002.

Hawkins, David R. *Power vs. Force: The Hidden Determinants of Human Behavior*. New York: Hay House, Inc., 1995.

Hill, Napoleon. *Think and Grow Rich*. Meriden, CT: The Ralston Society, 1937.

The Holy Bible, King James Version. Book of James. Grand Rapids: Zondervan Publishing House, 2010.

Martone, Jeff. *Kettlebell Rx: The Complete Guide for Athletes and Coaches*. Victory Belt Publishing, 2011.

Murphy, T. J. *Inside the Box: How CrossFit Shredded the Rules, Stripped Down the Gym, and Rebuilt My Body*. Boulder, CO: VeloPress, 2012.

Murphy, T. J. and Brian MacKenzie. *Unbreakable Runner: Unleash the Power of Strength and Conditioning for a Lifetime of Running Strong*. Boulder, CO: VeloPress, 2014.

Musashi, Miyamoto. *The Book of Five Rings*. Translated by William Scott Wilson. Boston: Shambhala Publications, Inc., 2002.

Rinpoche, Yongey Mingyur. *The Joy of Living: Unlocking the Secret and Science of Happiness*. New York: Harmony Books, 2007.

Sears, Barry. *Enter the Zone: A Dietary Road Map*. New York: HarperCollins Publishers, Inc., 1995.

Starrett, Kelly and T. J. Murphy. *Ready to Run: Unlocking Your Potential to Run Naturally*. Victory Belt Publishing, 2014.

Articles

Amundson, Greg. "The Chink in My Armor." *CrossFit Journal*. September 16, 2009. http://journal.crossfit.com/2009/09/the-chink-in-my-armor.tpl.

—. "Coaching the Mental Side of CrossFit." *CrossFit Journal*. July 7, 2010. http://journal.crossfit.com/2010/07/coaching-the-mental-side-of-crossfit.tpl.

—. "CrossFit HQ, 2851 Research Park Dr., Santa Cruz, Calif." *CrossFit Journal*. January 5, 2010. http://journal.crossfit.com/2010/01/crossfit-hq-2851-research-park-dr-santa-cruz-calif.tpl.

—. "Diet Secrets of the Tupperware Man." *CrossFit Journal*. December 29, 2008. http://journal.crossfit.com/2008/12/diet-secrets-of-the-tupperware-man.tpl.

—. "Diet Secrets of the Tupperware Man Vol. 2." *CrossFit Journal*. June 20, 2012. http://journal.crossfit.com/2012/06/diet-secrets-of-the-tupperware-man-vol-2.tpl.

—. "Forging Elite Leadership." *CrossFit Journal*. April 18, 2011. http://journal.crossfit.com/2011/04/forging-elite-leadership.tpl.

—. "Garage Gym 101: How to Grow a Successful Garage Gym." *CrossFit Journal*. February 20, 2010. http://journal.crossfit.com/2010/02/garage-gym-101-how-to-grow-a-successful-garage-gym.tpl.

—. "Training 2 Miles to Run 100." *CrossFit Journal*. February 19, 2009. http://journal.crossfit.com/2009/02/training-2-miles-to-run-100.tpl.

Online

www.crossfit.com

www.crossfitsantacruzcentral.com

www.mikesgym.org

Acknowledgments

My life has certainly been blessed with many wonderful mentors, incredible coaches, and dear friends. Therefore, the task of deciding whom to list in the acknowledgments section proved to be very challenging. First and foremost, I am grateful that I have come to intimately know God in my life. As I grow older and (hopefully) a bit wiser, I find that more and more of my day is filled with prayer and reflection on the wondrous Creator of all things.

I am also grateful for the life lessons my dad and mom taught me, even until moments before their deaths. On August 20, 2000, my dad was nearing the end of his battle with terminal cancer. With tears in my eyes, I stood at his bedside at Dameron Hospital in Stockton, California, and whispered in his ear, "Dad, I'm going to make you proud of me." He opened his eyes and smiled, and then, through a strained voice, he gently reminded me, "Son, whatever you do, do it for love."

My mom taught me to be willing and ready to forgo the comforts of life to help serve and encourage others. The final year of my mom's life was spent living in a small hut in a tiny village in Jordan, teaching and ministering to the poor and underprivileged village children. During her service as a Peace Corps volunteer in Jordan, she slept on the ground and all of her possessions fit into one small bag. Just hours before slipping into a coma she would never return from, my mother told me, "Greg, everybody can encourage somebody and be supported at the same time."

To my younger brothers, Erik, Stephen, and Mark, thank you for letting me be your "big brother" even though you are all much taller than me. You are my best friends.

I am grateful to all of the highly talented coaches who have had a profoundly positive influence on my life. Chief among them is Karen Glahan, my high school speech coach, who taught me the value of language and that public speaking is a skill of a warrior. Thanks to my athletic coaches, including the founder of CrossFit, "Coach" Greg Glassman, and my high school water polo coach, Scott McGregor. Both men taught me the value of dedicated training, and Greg inspired me to realize that the greatest adaptation to physical training is in fact mental. Coach Glassman also helped carry the torch of mentorship in my life following the death of my dad.

Thanks also to my martial arts and yoga instructors, including John "PIT Master" Hackleman; the legendary Brazilian jiu-jitsu black-belt instructor Garth Taylor; US Navy SEAL veteran and acclaimed author Mark Divine; and my mentors in Krav Maga, including Londale Theus, Kelly Campbell, Jon Pascal, Michael Margolin, and Tina Angelita. Collectively, I learned from these masters that force may overcome other people, but only power will overcome ourselves.

To the warriors I have served alongside, I am indebted to you now and always: Major Laverty, Captain Couchman, Captain Currie, Captain Hill, Captain Thomas, and Captain Sandervol of the US Army; to the Santa Cruz County Sheriff's Office, Scotts Valley Police Department, and Santa Cruz Harbor Patrol for providing an institution that fostered my warrior spirit; and the agents of the Drug Enforcement Administration and Border Enforcement Security Task Force team, whom I served with in Quantico, Virginia, and in the Imperial County District Office in Imperial County, California.

To my longtime friend and brilliant coauthor, T. J. Murphy, who believed in the message contained in this book, and a special thanks to the team at VeloPress, including Casey Blaine, Vicki Hopewell, and Kara Mannix. A great deal of gratitude is also extended to my agent Linda Konner for her terrific guidance and support.

Finally, to the athletes of the past, present, and future at CrossFit Amundson in Santa Cruz, California, for your help in building a gym and community that radiate fitness of the mind, body, and spirit.

About the Authors

Greg Amundson is an ecclesiastically endorsed and ordained minister, a thought leader in integrated wellness practices, and a prolific author and speaker whose message has positively influenced the lives of thousands of spiritual seekers. He is an alumnus of the University of California at Santa Cruz (BA in legal theory) and Western Theological Seminary (MA in leadership and MA in biblical and theological studies).

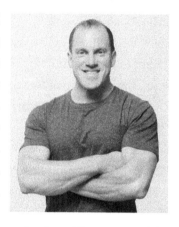

Greg also spent over 22 years in warrior professions. He was a captain in the United States Army, a Special Weapons and Tactics (SWAT) team operator and sniper in Santa Cruz, California, a special agent with the Drug Enforcement Administration (DEA), and the DEA liaison to the highly effective Border Enforcement Security Taskforce (BEST) team.

In addition to his extensive government service, Greg has dedicated years to mastering various disciplines. Greg founded the CrossFit® Goal Setting Course and CrossFit® Law Enforcement Application Course and was a former owner of the nation's first CrossFit® gym. For the past 20 years, Greg has traveled worldwide, teaching functional fitness and self-mastery principles. Greg is a Krav Maga black belt with Krav Maga Worldwide and the Krav Maga Association of America. He is also a "top gun" graduate of the Los Angeles Police Department's (LAPD) Handgun Instructor Training School (HITS). Greg is now a senior instructor at the Federal Law Enforcement Training Centers (FLETC) and the best-selling author of *The Warrior and the Monk* and *Fresh Wind*. To learn more or connect with Greg, visit www.gregoryamundson.com.

T. J. Murphy, NASM CPT, is a veteran journalist and editor who has coauthored two *New York Times* best sellers, *Unbreakable Runner*, with Brian MacKenzie, and *Ready to Run*, with Kelly Starrett. His feature writing has appeared in *Outside Magazine*, *Runner's World*, Spartan.com, and *Triathlete Magazine*. T. J. is a 2:38 marathoner who has finished five Ironmans. His first foray into writing about general 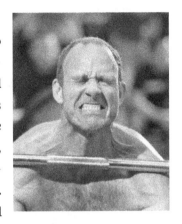 fitness was the book *Inside the Box: How CrossFit® Shredded the Rules, Stripped Down the Gym, and Rebuilt My Body*. T. J. lives in Boston with his wife, Gretchen, and their two kids, Milo and Maddie.